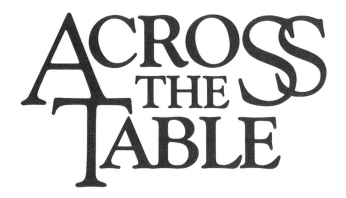

Across the Table

An Indulgent Look at Food in Canada

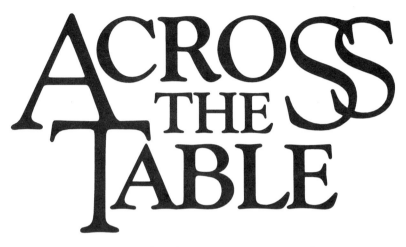

ACROSS THE TABLE

An Indulgent Look at Food in Canada

by Cynthia Berney Wine
Original Watercolours by
Mary Pratt

Prentice-Hall Canada Inc.
Scarborough, Ontario

Canadian Cataloguing in Publication Data

Wine, Cynthia.
Across the table: an indulgent look at food in Canada

ISBN 0-13-003641-2

1. Diet—Canada. 2. Cookery—Canada. 3. Food
habits—Canada. 4. Pratt, Mary, 1935–
5. Food in art. I. Pratt, Mary, 1935–
II. Title.

TX360.C3W56 1985   641.3'00971   C85-098846-2

Published by Prentice-Hall Canada Inc., Scarborough, Ontario

Prentice-Hall Inc., Englewood Cliffs, *New Jersey*
Prentice-Hall International, Inc., *London*
Prentice-Hall of Australia, Pty., Ltd., *Sydney*
Prentice-Hall of India Pvt., Ltd., *New Delhi*
Prentice-Hall of Japan, Inc., *Tokyo*
Prentice-Hall of Southeast Asia (Pte.) Ltd., *Singapore*
Editora Prentice-Hall do Brasil Ltda., *Rio de Janeiro*
Prentice-Hall Hispanoamericana, S.A., *Mexico*
Whitehall Books Ltd., Wellington, *New Zealand*

ISBN 0-13-003641-2

Editor: Shelley Tanaka
Production Editor: Clare Rundall
Production: Rand Paterson
Recipe Tester: Kathy Chute
Design: René Demers
Colour Separations: Herzig Somerville
Composition: Attic Typesetting Inc.

Printed and bound in Canada by The Bryant Press Limited

1 2 3 4 5 BP 89 88 87 86 85

To my children, Hayley and Joshua
—*Cynthia Wine*

To my children and grandchildren,
John, Anne, Barby,
Ned, Katherine and Elizabeth
—*Mary Pratt*

ACKNOWLEDGEMENTS

My thanks to *Homemaker's* magazine, which sponsored travels from 1980 to 1983, especially editor Jane Gale who with Mebbie Black and Ursula Kaiser provided years of encouragement and support.

Air Canada sponsored a further cross-country trip so I could collect new information for this book. This is a mammoth country, and I could not have travelled so freely without their help.

I cannot begin to list the people who took me home to mother or to their favourite chip stands. Only some of their names appear in this book. Restaurateurs were always very helpful, letting me poke in their kitchens and ask odd questions about what made their food taste good. Thank you all.

Others spent hours across tables telling me what to eat in their areas and providing me with much information about food in Canada. Some of them are mentioned in the copy. To name them all is impossible, though I wish I could. Among them are Julian Armstrong, Elizabeth Baird, Mme Jehanne Benoit, Ada and Martin Berney, Carole and Sheldon Berney, Willy Brand, Trudi and Lester Clements, Alison Cumming, Judy and Alan Comfort, Hilda Fauchon, Jack Ferry, Betty Fitzsimmons, Francie and Ken Frank, Joanne Good, James Gray, Paul and Audrey Grescoe, Marion Holler, Mechtild Hoppenrath, Marg Kearney, Dinah Koo, Suzanne Leclerc, Anne Lindsay, Marilyn Linton, Bee Macguire, Florence Manor, Susan Mendelson, Sheila Moore, Karen Neal, Butch Nepon, Marie Nightingale, Charles Oberdorf, Peter Puxley, Bill and Elizabeth Raine, Judy Schultz, Gail Singer, Bonnie Stern, Ronnie and Barry Tessler, Marion Warhaft and Lucy Waverman. Others corrected and commented as I wrote, among them Ford Clements and Sheila Kieran.

Shelley Tanaka edited this book with thoroughness, unmuddling the muddled and shining up the paragraphs to make a five-year diary digestible.

Kathy Chute tested all the recipes in her home in Nova Scotia and provided much advice on how to make good things taste even better.

There have been many involved in the concept and production of this book. Thanks to Nancy Colbert of the Colbert Agency Inc. who with Denise Schon and Jan Whitford initiated this project, and to Iris Skeoch, Clare Rundall and others at Prentice-Hall Canada who carried it through.

I am especially grateful to Mary Pratt who gave her considerable talent to this project and to Christopher Pratt who made our meetings so much fun.

And last, but always first, I am grateful to my family, who have endured meals of muktuk and miles of sausages when I was too busy to prepare the hot beef sandwiches they really wanted.

—*Cynthia Wine*

Mira Godard and Philip Ottenbrite of the Mira Godard Gallery in Toronto were unceasingly cooperative and provided invaluable advice.

Christopher endured a summer of sailing with no cook in the galley.

—*Mary Pratt*

LIST OF WATERCOLOURS

TABLE OF CONTENTS

PREFACE

S it a group of hungry people across a table with a good meal in front of them, and chances are they'll start talking about the wonderful dinner they had the night before. This book is the result of five years of such conversations, and the meals that created them.

The treasures that I found were due to the people who enthusiastically directed me to their favourite private kitchens, restaurants and roadside stands. Most were strangers who happily told me what they ate, then took me home to prove how good it was. Boy, was it good.

I was enormously grateful for such eaters, because sometimes my travels were plagued by Canadians who were on austere regimens or who argued through every mouthful that they should be. But, thankfully, the Canadian appetite is not on a diet. And the Canadian appetite is not homogeneous. Once I got away from the mass-produced technological foods that are the same everywhere in the western world, I found differences that form the basis of the six regions in this book. And there were things I could count on everywhere. We have wonderful breakfasts in Canada; we also have good baking. Nearly everywhere our pies (especially berry pies), buns and breads can't be rivalled, a legacy perhaps from all the years when the stove heating the house served double use to bake all day.

The best food in the country is to be found in private homes, often hidden from the rest of us. Sometimes the dishes have been in the family for years, like the coconut cake that Mary Darcy made in Newfoundland, or the griddle cakes Tony Pistun's sister made in Saskatoon. Sometimes the dishes are more modern, like the paper-thin salmon with horseradish and mustard sauce that an Edmonton man made when I called to ask what was up for dinner.

I was as grateful for the company and advice as I was for the food. I was away from my own table for two or three weeks at a time, and I found the commonality created by food very comforting. So was the advice. I was sent to favourite restaurants and warned away from others. I was cautioned about the woman in Prince Edward Island who sometimes slips skim milk into her lobster chowder. In Alberta a listener phoned an open-line show I was on to warn me about the huge amounts of food I would be served in the local restaurants. She reported that her personal survey had revealed that the number of doggie bags leaving Calgary eateries exceeded the canine population by eighty-five percent.

As I travelled, people would often refer to the stunning paintings of everyday food by Newfoundland artist Mary Pratt. I had seen *Red Currant Jelly*, which hangs in the National Gallery, and had marvelled at the explicit richness of *Salmon on Saran* and *Baked Apples in Tinfoil*. But it was the reports of Mary's oatmeal bread—which she bakes, not paints—that prompted me to call her in 1981 and ask if I could come for lunch. She served the oatmeal bread and a wonderful concoction her family calls health soup. And, like Canadians everywhere, she talked of other meals. "Think of the bowl of porridge a child sits down to at breakfast. The white cream surrounds the hot island of oatmeal. The brown sugar melts into it. Oh, it's beautiful stuff. Or a simple china bowl filled with white sugar. Just picture it! When the light hits the sugar, the sugar shimmers. The spoon resting on the sugar makes a soft dent. The sight of it is so nostalgic, so evocative, but with such wonderful texture. I never see it anywhere else."

It seemed too much to hope that Mary would join this project, but she did, so I had another chance to visit her home—this time for a fabulous meat pie, with apple cobbler for dessert. I tell you about the meals, because the paintings speak for themselves.

I received much help from Canada's professional eaters—a group of food writers that has increased in size and weight with the growing interest in food in this country. Eating for a living is not without its hazards. This is an overfed bunch who, when offered caviar for a first course and fresh scallops with raspberry vinaigrette for the second, are likely to groan, "Oh, no, not again." For the years I was a member of that tribe, we attended press conferences and watched cooks create odd mosaics at chefs' competitions. We stood aghast one year in Frankfurt, Germany, as a Canadian chef won first prize for a montage of an Indian chief's head he'd created from marzipan and olives, then arranged on the rump of a pig. We sat politely through a luncheon organized to promote an artificial sweetener, where the stuff had been incorporated into every one of the five courses.

Then one day I heard about a man who had found a way to combine mashed pumpkin with pasta. He was seriously described to me as a man of vision. It was, in fact, later that week, when a representative of the fruit industry in the United States signed his letter, "Cherrily Yours," that I began to want to go home. This book is about all the good things I ate before I did.

Sometimes food reporters in Canada sense a general feeling of inadequacy about the food we have here—a sort of edible complex. This is completely insupportable. We have wonderful food in Canada. We just don't let it show as much as folks in other countries do.

I hope this book will begin to redress the balance.

Cynthia Berney Wine
Toronto
September, 1985

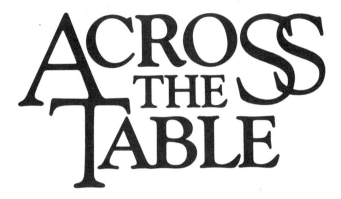

An Indulgent Look at
Food in Canada

INTRODUCTION

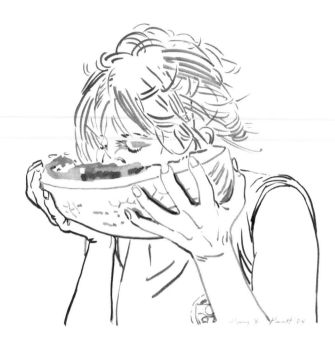

Canada is over one hundred years old, and by now you'd think we would have come up with a national dish—something we could call our own, so we don't have to borrow hot dogs on July 1 or turkey on Thanksgiving.

A visitor to Canada from one of those countries that's smug about its cuisine, told me once that the dish he met most often in roadside diners was brown meat on white bread with gravy. We have the world's most succulent beef and even the Russians envy our wheat. How did we manage to turn them into the hot beef sandwich?

What's worse is that visitors to Canada often get the impression that there's nothing much better to chew on here. I have gained eleven new pounds eating across Canada, and not one is owed to the hot beef sandwich. Those pounds are in place because of lobster chowder made with cream in Prince Edward Island, fresh cod baked in cheese sauce in Newfoundland, maple bread spread with salt pork in Quebec, basil bread in Whitehorse and cinnamon buns sticky with glazed sugar and sweet butter in Manitoba.

As I travelled across the country, within each area I found foods I'd never heard of. When they were especially good, I wondered why. At my first taste of cod in cheese in Newfoundland, triple-crust blueberry pie near the Bay of Chaleur or bannock baked light and flaky in Whitehorse, I wondered how I could have lived so many years next to these dishes without knowing what I was missing. We know more about the food of northern Italy.

The Canadian stomach, it seems, doesn't travel in Canada. Nationality is a political concept, not a gastronomic one. Our good food tends to stay put in the regions of Canada, and our eating regions are very distinct. Both British Columbia and the Atlantic provinces have fish, but they are prepared differently in each area. Even within regions there are regions. In Newfoundland where they combine salt cod and potatoes to make fish 'n brewis (pronounced "bruise") they know nothing of Dutch Mess, a dish of the same ingredients that tastes completely different when it's made in Lunenburg, Nova Scotia.

Canada's regional food has developed as incoming peoples adapt the local produce to their own dishes. In Liverpool, Nova Scotia, Jimmy Sapp, whose family is from Lebanon, mixed cold cooked fresh lobster with lemon juice and garlic for a lobster salad that knocks your socks off and is heresy to the Atlantic Canadians who have always mixed it with cream, if anything. Gail Singer from Winnipeg makes cabbage rolls from caribou meat. If she has a whole roast of caribou, she serves it with couscous. At the Italian cultural centre in Toronto, the specialty in the cafeteria has been bacon on a bagel.

Nationalists who wish to promote a coast-to-coast cuisine have a rough road to travel. Gastronomic regions flow south to north rather than east to west. Our regional food is more likely to be influenced by the United States than another Canadian province. That's especially true in the cities. If you want to know what they'll be eating at chic parties next year in Vancouver, look at what they are eating at chic parties this year in Los Angeles and San Francisco. In Toronto, keep an eye on New York. In the Atlantic provinces the cookbooks of traditional local recipes are full of dishes like those put out by groups in Maine. And for local specialties, look at the people who have settled in the areas. Sauerkraut is big in Lunenburg and in Kitchener, Ontario, because of the German influence. Three-crust pies are eaten both in Quebec and New Brunswick because they're made by the French Canadians who settled in both places.

And within different regions and different cities, there is also the unexpected. Vancouver has great chocolate. Montreal has good junk food. Middle-eastern donairs (pita stuffed with shaved meat and topped with spicy-sweet sauce) are as common as hamburgers in Nova Scotia and New Brunswick. When that happens, it's usually the local immigration that's made the difference. Vancouver has wonderful chocolate because a couple of good chocolate-makers settled there and now anyone else who makes chocolate must meet their standards. Calgary has some of the best tandoori chicken in Canada—not because of the geography or climate, or even because of its chickens—but because Inderjit Singh, who knows how to fix a terrific tandoori chicken, moved to Calgary from Singapore to be near his brother and opened the Moti Mahal restaurant.

If we're culinary strangers to one another, food merchants all over the world know and cherish what we offer. Frieda who imports and distributes exotic foods throughout the United States wants fiddleheads. Everyone wants wild rice and maple syrup. Arctic char is big. The fancy food shops in New York take our Ontario Cheddar, our peameal bacon and sometimes our Malpeque oysters. One place imports prosciutto ham made in Ontario and sells it as Italian. Businessmen love to take Canadian whisky back to Japan.

I once watched a boatload of freshly caught squid leaving an Atlantic dock for Boston. Our salted cod goes to the Caribbean; our herring roe to Japan. It will be argued that these losses have as much to do with international politics and pricing as they do with Canadian tastes and other issues that deserve a book of their own, but wouldn't it be great to have a dish of local calamari—fried fast and rained with fresh lemon juice—in Halifax? Imagine how it would taste with a glass of chilled Atlantic beer.

Our official concern with defining a Canadian cuisine began at our centenary in 1967, when Canadian chefs, most of whom had been trained in Europe, scrambled to collect the dishes we would show to the world. The first official handbook published by the Canadian Federation of Chefs de Cuisine promised that fiddlehead soup, marinated buffalo and poached British Columbia salmon were genuinely Canadian. But identifying national dishes has remained primarily a preoccupation of chefs and politicians. Food as a statement of our culture doesn't show in our public pursuits. The highways into our cities are lined with corporate fast food places; the restaurants that reflect local produce and local culinary aspirations are always out of the way and hard to find. And Ottawa's Parliamentary dining room (only MPs, their guests, senior staff and members of the press are allowed to order at its hallowed, tax-supported tables) hardly sets a sterling example. Most Canadians applauded a recent move to raise the cost of a meal to $8 from $4.40—a response that totally ignores the fact that, even at $4.40, guests were overcharged for the

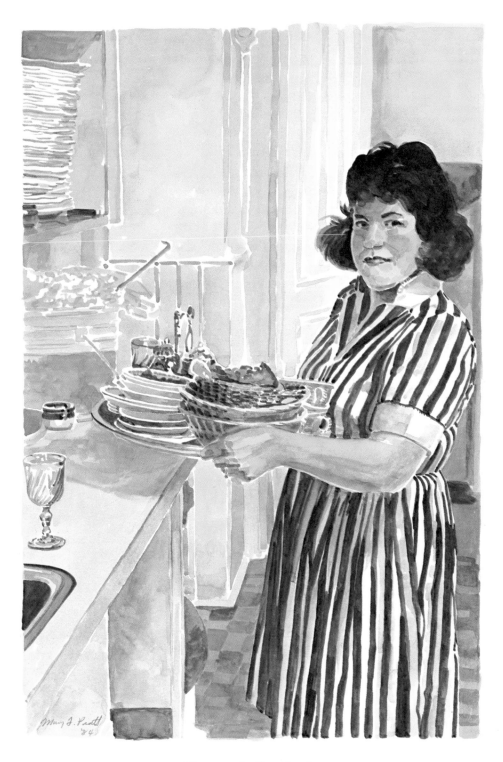

Waitress at the Blomidon Inn

restaurant's flannelly meats, flaccid vegetables and air-dried cheese.

After official banquets and convention dinners, unwary visitors tend to leave our country with the impression that we exist on overdone beef and mountains of mashed. Even the "official" Canadian meal of salmon, fiddleheads, wild rice and maple mousse—a meal that's wonderful when it's prepared for four people—can be a disaster when slung for hundreds. Wild rice can survive almost anything, but fresh salmon and fiddleheads tend to suffer from mass production.

One reason Canadians are not traditionally food conscious is that food wasn't uppermost in pioneers' minds. Keeping warm was. Someone has estimated that it takes four thousand calories to work a day outdoors in the cold. You don't get four thousand calories from kiwi—you get it from hot beef sandwiches, from tourtière, from dense bread spread thick with pork fat and from French fries afloat in gravy. People who work outdoors today know that, too. The Canadian team that climbed Mount Everest were offered anything they wanted to eat. Did they ask for sushi and bean sprouts? They asked for—and got—Christmas cake (with suet and brandy), Mars bars and chile con carne.

To appreciate the foods that are traditional throughout the regions of Canada, you must have an appreciation of fat. It's customary to think that fat keeps you warm and, in the rural parts of this country, you still hear people saying that you need some fat on you for the winter. Traditionally, you ate what you could in the fall and stored as much as possible, in the basement and on the body. (A Canadian psychologist who deals with eating disorders once told me that the average Canadian still puts on eight pounds of fat every winter.) Even today, Canadians have a hoarding mentality about food. As a Mexican woman living in Toronto said, "Canadians are so insecure about food. They feel they have to store it and make sure they always have lots—in freezers, refrigerators and cupboards. In Mexico, people just eat a meal. There are no leftovers."

Whatever produce we had was made fuel intensive. Even foods that were naturally lean were fattened. Fish was coated in batter and fried in fat; beef and berries were encased in pastry. Early Canadians baked as much as they could because wood fuel was cheap and heated the kitchen while it cooked the dinner.

All that fat may add to our difficulties in defining a Canadian cuisine. Today's eaters, conscious of calorie consumption and the world's food fads, find the dishes that are traditional to the regions of Canada unfashionable for these lean times.

These days, our appetites are threatened by an almost pathological phobia about fat. We loathe the stuff—on our bodies and on our plates. The price of this phobia may be some of Canada's best dishes. We're suspicious of the cream and canned milk that sustain the Atlantic chowders. We distrust the crusts on Quebec's tourtière and cipaille; the smoked juicy sausages of the Prairies. To understand Canadian food, you have to have some feeling for the pleasures of fat foods. In my travels across Canada, some of the best things I ate were liberally dosed with fat: sweetbread pâté that consisted of half sweetbreads and half butter, salt pork spread on maple bread, marrow from a soup stock spread on black bread. And airport breakfasts of bacon and eggs with white bread soaked in far too much salty yellow butter.

The simple foods we now love, full of flavour but low in fat, are the luxury of a society whose members drive home from the office to sit in centrally heated buildings. The variety we now demand on our menus, in our institutions or at home is partly the result of security and abundance. It's easy for us to play with new foods now—there's always something else to eat if we don't like them. But our ancestors ate what was put in front of them.

We had little use for spices and odd herbs in our early days of settlement. Then, just getting three square meals a day was culinary adventure enough. In other countries, spices were often used to help preserve foods; but in Canada we had our cool root cellars and, in winter, the world was our freezer.

For years, our lack of familiarity with spices and our suspicion that strange-tasting foods and culinary exotica were somehow contrary to the democratic spirit, bequeathed us a legacy of distrust for odd flavours. Food was for function, not fun. Overattention to the pleasures of the palate was contrary to Puritan sensibilities. There was something just a mite subversive about folks who could flaunt their fresh fennel, who spent time and money on their stomachs instead of their souls.

There might have been some respite from this thin-lipped mistrust in the waves of immigration into Canada in the early part of this century, when the nearly four hundred thousand newcomers brought a great variety of gastronomic backgrounds. There were also new-fangled appliances to make food preparation easier: iceboxes, electric stoves and co-op food stores were becoming known.

But, just as the chance came to taste new foods and recognize that perfectly nice people ate spices, two wars and a Depression took away our appetites. The awakening had to wait until the 1960s, when finally we were affluent and secure enough to begin experimenting with funny foods. After more than twenty years of travelling abroad, we had discovered that it was possible and even desirable to eat a dish flavoured with oregano. And even if we didn't travel, we watched television cooking shows that showed us beef Wellington and Black Forest cake.

Although we began to sample dishes from other cuisines, we weren't curious to find out what else there was to eat in Canada. What we have discovered about one another has been as much an accident of technology and advances in transportation as it has been purposeful demand. Thirty years ago fresh salmon was a true exotic in Manitoba. Today people can sit at tables in Winnipeg and debate the merits of Atlantic salmon over Pacific.

The back-to-the-land movement of the sixties taught us to reject any additives or food that wasn't pure. It also fostered our distrust of meat and our worship of fresh fruits and vegetables. The generation in Canada that had learned to cook from soothing Kraft television commercials in the fifties ("just add one package of Kraft miniature marshmallows to one cup of Miracle Whip") abruptly turned its back on anything that came from a package. People began to live on farms and bake their own bread. If it had the space, the generation that had been raised on canned and frozen produce began to grow its own vegetables, or to fall out of bed at 6 a.m. on dark mornings to be the first at the city marketplace to pick over brown eggs.

Back to the earth gave way, in the seventies, to the wildest excesses of food madness. People collected cookbooks, cooking-class diplomas, gadgets and experiences. (I was once at a dinner party where eight people sat, enthralled, while our host described how he had rescued a lobster vol au vent from curdling by quickly stirring in an ice cube.) I can take you to a cupboard in my basement that is a graveyard for artichoke dishes, fondue forks, crockpots and melt-makers. My most briefly used gadget was an electric hot dog maker that electrocuted the sausage with a charge so intense that the lights dimmed in the house as each wiener met its maker.

People took classes as much to learn how to eat as to learn how to cook. It had become important to understand how a real trifle should taste and to know whether white or red wine should be served with veal. I learned of one woman who had attended over forty kinds of classes, all over the world. Another had a cookbook collection of over three hundred books. (Incidentally, possibly the largest collection of cookbooks in the country belongs to the Niagara Falls, Ontario, regional library. It was bequeathed by the late Judy LaMarsh, one of Canada's best cooks.)

Now in the eighties, the fitness phenomenon and perhaps just plain fatigue has diminished the food frenzy. Enrolment in cooking classes is down, with exercise classes taking their place. The bathroom has overtaken the kitchen as the room in the house to decorate. Our interest in the culinary arts has remained high, but it's now centred on wine and restaurants and take-out as much as it once was on home cooking. Today people collect bakery croissants and eating-out experiences the way they collected stereo equipment a couple of decades ago. We dart from one restaurant to another—a different one every night—in a kind of gastronomic promiscuity, afraid to become too intimate with one, lest it reduce our desire to experience another.

Nonetheless, we are foraging for food in a way that would have earned a belly laugh from our ancestors who left their native lands for Canada just so they could avoid getting up at dawn to collect fresh eggs. Now we check labels and boil vegetables in Perrier. We go to great lengths and expense for fresh water. Near Toronto, on Mississauga Road north of the Queensway and south of Dundas, is a pipe that brings spring water to those willing to make the drive to get it. There are Sundays when you have to wait in line.

Today we expect food to be an experience. We want crunch and contrast, colour and light. We want fibre and pulp for roughage and tomato peel roses for our sensibilities.

At first, the fitness phenomenon took the strongest hold in our cities; for awhile we could count on the folks in the country to keep the faith in fat alive. But even there, people now huddle in farmhouses to discuss the latest fibre cereal. In town the businessman who once could be counted on to order steak at lunch has been converted. He used to love steak because it was so masculine and because it was an easy thing to order when his mind was really on bottom lines. Cute menus offering carrot and ginger soup were a distraction from scribbling numbers on placemats. Now the same guy orders the abalone with a white wine spritzer for lunch—unless he's planning to make it for supper.

The granola gurus have won. Fashionable Canadians who live in a nation that is cold most of the year eat summer food year-round. We purée spinach and serve it in a splat on a white plate with a piece of poached fish and a carrot cut into a tulip. We sprinkle raw bran on yoghurt and sip herbal teas, decaffeinated coffees (Swiss-water method) or even hot water with lemon juice. Some of this is just fashion—the Chianti bottle with a dripping candle has been replaced in restaurants by a Perrier bottle with a daisy—but some is an excessive concern with health.

We carefully watch each other to see how we're doing. When an obese man lowered himself into a chair in a Vancouver restaurant, the woman next to me gasped, "My God, he's going to eat again." It was all she could do not to lean over and offer him some advice on fitness and nutrition. We've traded the Victorian hatred of the sin of lust for our own revulsion at the sin of gluttony. As a university professor pointed out, "After all, gluttony is the sin you can see." Overweight people are to be abhorred and converted or simply abhorred and ignored.

One of the peculiar results of our feeling about food is found in some of our food writing and advertising, with its emphasis on transposing phrases from the bedroom to the dining room. Sauces are "silken," a dish is "kissed" by a herb, we "yearn" for a salad. Try asking your date if he'll have whipped cream on his custard. His shocked reply may be "I don't do that sort of thing."

And restaurants play along with our food-as-lust fantasies. Chocolate and whipped cream is called Divine Decadence in a spiffy Vancouver dining room and, in Calgary, there's a place that offers Better-Than-Sex Squares. (They may be, but frankly, who wants to know?) A rich dessert in a Toronto restaurant frequented by the kiss-kiss crowd is called Death by Chocolate.

But the food frenzy of the seventies permanently changed Canadians, giving us a raised consciousness about food and a sophistication about eating that this country's pioneers might have decried as indulgent. We now have a group of fine cooks, some of whom have parlayed their own interest into catering. Not only have they turned their own interest into a livelihood; they have done wonders for those people who couldn't care less about cooking but are under pressure to keep up. Now good eating is as much a matter of knowing where to shop as knowing how to cook.

The lady next door who makes fabulous spaghetti sauce begins to bottle it; her neighbour down the block who has a great recipe for pâté or cheesecake offers it to food shops or restaurants. Sable and Rosenfeld, two Toronto women who mixed up their first batch of grandmother's mustard in a pink plastic baby's bathtub, now distribute it all over the world. Everyone wonders whether their treasured family recipes are saleable. Some of them are. You can pay eight dollars for a terrific chocolate cake in a downtown store which was made by your neighbour. In less competitive days you might have had it for free with a cup of coffee.

Today, professional Canadian chefs enjoy an excellent reputation among their international colleagues. Canada has done spectacularly well at the Kosher Culinary Olympics in Israel. In the last decade we have distinguished ourselves at the International Culinary Olympics in Frankfurt. In 1976 we'd placed second in the world and, four years later, our national team placed third after Germany and the United States, while a team from British Columbia came home laden with gold and silver. In 1984 a team from Toronto swept every division it entered, capturing five gold medals, one grand gold and two special awards. Our chefs won with their thirty-one distinctive platters of caribou, salmon, mussels, lobster, scallops and fiddleheads—foods we all applaud as being distinctively Canadian.

We are finally discovering foods that are wonderful to eat in Canada. But we are keeping many more dishes a secret in our own regions. They are at their best in their own homes, surrounded by people who love them. You can't homogenize regional cooking. When you try to force-feed a national cuisine, you get abominations like the halibut in maple syrup once promoted by a fish company anxious for Canadian content, or the Canadian Caesar, a drink made of spiced clamato juice and whisky that I once ordered at the Toronto airport.

We don't need a national dish and heaven spare us from a national drink. The very lack of them expresses the diversity we have. The Canadian larder is divided into regions—each stuffed to overflowing with foods that can bring us as close to gastronomic heaven as we are likely to get. Find fish that has been cooked fresh and flaking in the East, or berry pies that squirt bright juice at first bite in the North. You can't eat better anywhere.

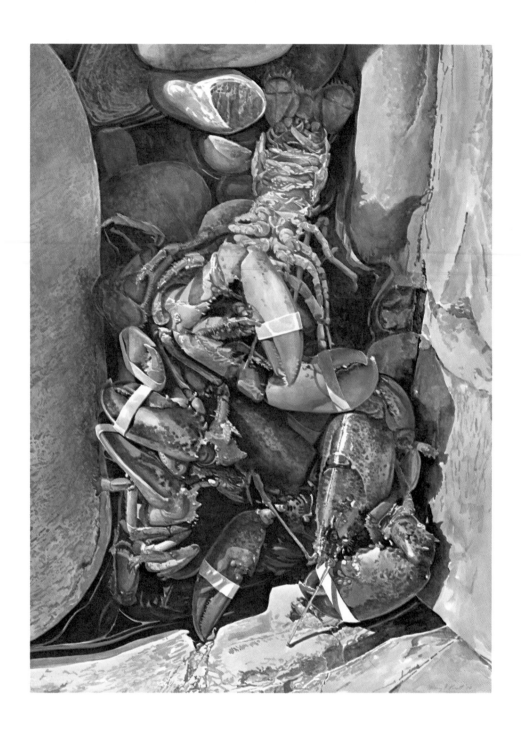

Live lobsters with claw bands

*A creature bound and ready for the pot is a sobering
vision, even if the creature is, according to scientists,
"just a large and rather tasty insect." (M.P.)*

THE ATLANTIC PROVINCES

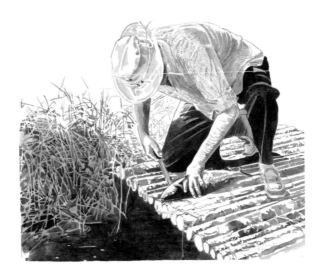

No one in Canada clings to the food of childhood with the tenacity of people from Atlantic Canada.

Before I ever went to Atlantic Canada, I met its food in the delicious stories and hungry reminiscences of people who had grown up there. They had left for better jobs and worse dinners in other parts of the country and now seemed condemned to spend their leisure time waxing rhapsodic about the scrunchions and grape-nuts ice cream they had left behind.

What is it about the food of the East, that grown people cannot bear to be without it? If Manitobans can lead meaningful lives without pickerel cheeks, why can't Newfoundlanders carry on without cod's tongues?

The best of Atlantic food is a mystery to the rest of us. It even sounds foreign—figgy-duff, scrunchions, Dutch mess, hodge podge. And when you can make some sense out of part of the dish, the rest is a bafflement. How would you know that blueberry grunt was hot wild blueberries steamed with sweet dumplings and served with fresh cream? And what about the name would make you want to find out? There are a few Atlantic foods that we understand very well—lobster, Digby scallops, oysters from Prince Edward Island. Some of the drinks, like Newfie screech, are even better known; everybody everywhere knows about Maritime beer, and if you go to the right parties in Prince Edward Island, you'll know about potato vodka, too.

The other foods aren't easy to find, even when you're in the Atlantic provinces. It wasn't until I had lived there for months that I began to discover the local specialties and have an inkling of the extent of the underground Atlantic table.

That's because the best of Atlantic foods—in fact, the only Atlantic foods worth eating—are made in private homes, and it took that long before people would feed me what they actually ate themselves. In fact, they needed some convincing that that's what I wanted. People in Atlantic Canada are very shy about their food when they're on home territory. Take them out of their province and you hear about nothing else. But ask them who's a great cook when you're there, and they'll send you down the road to someone who has taken a Cordon Bleu course and "cooks fancy."

The foods of Atlantic Canada remain a mystery because they are rarely eaten by outsiders who can pass on the good news. The main reason for this is that travellers usually have to eat in restaurants, which are crummy at home cooking, not surprisingly. And home cooking in Atlantic Canada is superb.

Imagine the difference between a hot dog roasted over a fire and one grilled in a restaurant? That's the difference between salmon steak in a restaurant and a whole fresh Atlantic salmon splayed and tethered to an oak plank before it's faced to an open flame and grilled until its juices run sweet and buttery.

It's also hard to find good scrunchions in fancy eateries. These crisp renderings of salt pork flavour Atlantic concoctions like Newfoundland's fish n' brewis and Nova Scotia's Dutch mess. Commercial attempts at Dutch mess (a sumptuous concoction of salt cod, cream, potatoes and crunchy scrunchions) are as disappointing as overcooked corporate clams.

Hodge podge is one of the best examples of an Atlantic Canada dish that you can only get in homes. You can only have it once or twice a year because it is based on the produce of a garden at its peak, in a region that doesn't enjoy fresh vegetables during most of the year. You take fresh peas from the garden, shell them fast and throw them into a pot. On top of that toss freshly dug new potatoes, washed but not scrubbed to maintain their snappy skin.

Then carrots, left whole, yellow and green beans and lots of new onions. Add some water and boil it all together fast, so the flavours all blend together and bits of onion stick to the carrot and pieces of potato skin join the new potatoes. When the potatoes are tender, drain the vegetables and toss them with lots of the freshest butter you can find. And don't worry if the carrots and peas are not al dente. This is a vegetable dish of a different order. When it's all mixed together and glistening with butter in a huge bowl, you take fresh cream (the kind you have to get by knocking on Mrs. Henderson's back door in Brooklyn, Nova Scotia—not that washed out 35 percent supermarket cream) and pour lots of it over the hot vegetables. The cream gets warm and thick from the heat of the vegetables, and the vegetables get soft, almost mushy on the outside, but you can still bite through them in the centre. You have to eat hodge podge with a spoon so you don't miss any of that warm, sweetly vegetable-flavoured cream. There are variations, of course. Liz Raine likes to prepare a bowl of melted butter filled with garlic and drizzle that on top, as if there isn't enough butter and cream in that dish to carry a coureur du bois through January.

Fortunately for their cuisine, past generations of Atlantic Canadians didn't suffer the horror of fat that plagues us today. Cream, butter and fried foods have been fundamental to their diets, if not to their philosophy. That's why cost-efficient restaurants can never duplicate the taste of the real stuff. No wonder tourists served a weak chowder, insipid with low-fat milk and margarine, wonder what all the fuss is about.

In Atlantic Canada, fat, on the plates and on the bodies, is a part of life. People still say in the fall that you need a little more fat on you to see you through the winter. Of course, some people have taken this rationale to extremes. Ned Mahanney in Wolfeville, Nova Scotia, used to remove the icing from a piece of cake, butter the cake and replace the icing. In homemade chowders, an extra dollop of butter is traditionally added to the bowl before the soup is ladled in. Atlantic chowder just isn't Atlantic chowder unless there are golden globules floating on top.

The best lobster chowder takes it one step further. The lobster meat is fried in butter before it is added to the potatoes, onions and canned milk, and maybe cream is added to that. The real strawberry shortcake is made with tea biscuits and lots of heavy whipped cream; in Newfoundland desserts are afloat in a stunning butter sauce. In Prince Edward Island you can find thick, clotted Devonshire cream. In New Brunswick there's a three-crust blueberry pie, so rich with pastry and packed with calories that it's reminiscent of the multi-crusted cipaille that kept Quebec's habitants warm through the winters.

Atlantic Canadians not only keep their superb dishes secret from the rest of Canada; they are also kept secret from each other. The Dutch mess so common in Lunenburg County in Nova Scotia is unheard of in Newfoundland, as foreign as cod au gratin (cod baked in a creamy cheese sauce) is to a person from Cape Breton. Although all the provinces have in

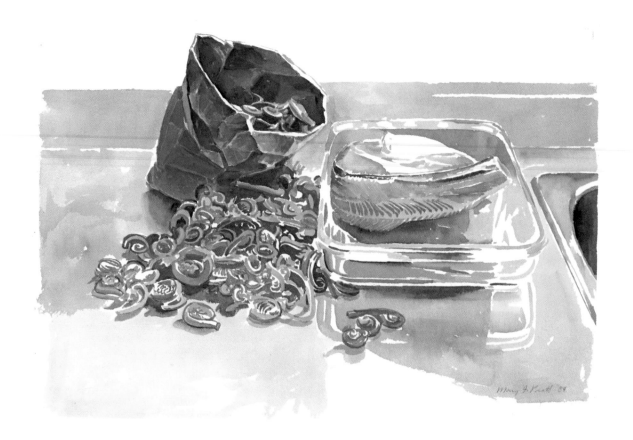

Fiddleheads and frozen salmon

*The pink of the fish and the moss green of the
fiddleheads always remind me of spring. I can even
smell the damp-woodsy smell of the little ferns mixed
with the sour smell of the wet paper bag. (M.P.)*

common in their cookery fish, fat and potatoes, the execution in each area is often unique.

Acadian specialties, for example, may be found throughout New Brunswick, along the French shore of Nova Scotia and in parts of Newfoundland. Probably the best known dish is pâté à la rapure or rappy pie, a gooey, wonderful dish made with grated potatoes, lots of salty grated onions and chicken, all topped with crumbly salt pork before it's baked.

In Prince Edward Island I prefer to take my quota of maritime fat in the form of Devonshire cream, a legacy of the province's British heritage. I take it with tea, which, in the island's private homes, is boiled to the point of blackness, and preserves made from the strawberries grown juicier and sweeter there than anywhere outside the Ile d'Orléans in Quebec. At mealtimes in Prince Edward Island you can't escape potatoes, served in every conceivable form, including a knockout potato chocolate cake.

The United Empire Loyalists from the United States brought many traditions like baked beans; the Scots who settled in Nova Scotia brought a love of baking. Round bake stones used for oatcakes can still be found in some kitchens and oatmeal is the cornerstone of baking throughout the Atlantic provinces.

The Germans who settled around the Lunenburg area in Nova Scotia were experts at pickling and preserving foods, so there you'll find the spicy Lunenburg sausage and its famous cousin, Lunenburg pudding. A slice of Lunenburg pudding rich with herbs with a smear of molasses is better than any of those fancy restaurant pâtés with their Cumberland sauces.

If fish, potatoes and fat are synonymous with survival throughout the Atlantic provinces, so is rum. The best known Atlantic rum is the Newfie screech now legal and a mere shadow of its original. The first screech was a thick, heavy rum brought from British Guyana by fishing crews. In Newfoundland the rum was diluted, bottled and sold for fifty cents for thirteen ounces. The drink was cheap and effective and became a great favourite with members of the Royal Canadian Navy. When a superior questioned the odd behaviour of his men, he was told, "It's that drink, sir. We drink it, walk a block, run a block and then screech a block." The name stuck, though the drink changed. Now the rum is imported from Jamaica and is quite respectable.

Like fat, rum in Atlantic Canada has some medicinal justifications. In Nova Scotia and New Brunswick, a cold cure for children is to stand them in a large dish of hot rum and let them inhale the curative fumes. I think hot rum is more fun when it works from the inside. To make a rum toddy, pour a generous measure of rum into a large mug. Fill the cup with boiling water. Flavour with honey and cinnamon stick. Drink slowly while wrapped in a wool blanket.

One of the myths about food in the Atlantic provinces is the notion that lobster is freely and constantly available. But lobster isn't as accessible as one might think. Fishing seasons are carefully controlled and monitored. On Nova Scotia's south shore, it used to be illegal to fish for lobster on a Sunday—even during the lobster season—because it was felt that the fisherman who went to church shouldn't be penalized for the lost fishing time.

People in Atlantic Canada love lobster, and they'll eat it a couple of times a year at home with family and friends. It is mostly cooked in seaweed and seawater, which gives Atlantic Canadians a slight edge on lobster cooked anywhere else, no matter how fresh it is. Willy Brand, former head of George Brown Cooking School in Toronto, considers the seawater steaming of live lobster to be a special Canadian technique. Some people have their own secrets. One man adds a bottle of beer to the pot, while another is horrified at the thought of disturbing the purity of the natural ingredients. "If you must have beer with the lobster," he sniffs, "put the beer in you and leave the pot alone."

These experts in Atlantic Canada know a great deal about lobster. They eat just about every part, except the yucky stuff in the head, but including the tomalley and liver and especially the succulent little nuggets cloistered where the legs meet the body. But whatever the ritual and with whatever expertise the lobster is consumed, it's not a frequent feast. "It's too rich to eat all the time," they'll tell you.

Despite its reputation as a luxury food now, lobster was once thought to be the baloney of the Atlantic—poor man's food, for families who could afford nothing better. People will tell stories of how they used to try to trade their lobster sandwiches at school for almost anything else, especially baloney. In New Brunswick parents were once not allowed to give their children lobster sandwiches more than twice a week.

But however often lobsters are served, where they're served seems to count more. Lobsters just don't taste right in restaurants, though that may be because Atlantic restaurants often overcook them and reduce their gentle insides to sharp chards. Lobsters taste better at home.

One of the reasons for this is that lobsters are ugly creatures with industrial-strength security systems. Achieving a chew of a lobster's insides is a task best performed in private with armaments commonly used for a gangland rumble. So it's best to eat them in private where you can relax and dismember. The kitchen table is swept clean of everything—salt

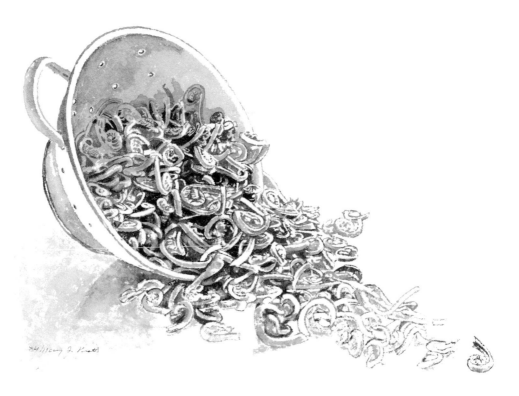

Fiddleheads from Harrison Farms

and pepper shakers, sugar bowl, Tonka trucks—and covered with yesterday's newspaper. The lobsters are tossed into the middle of the table, their red-hot armour is ravaged and their white meat trailed through melted butter or cider vinegar. You don't need to eat anything else with this feast—not French fries, not corn and certainly not salad or bread. You should occupy your hands and appetite with nothing but the wonderful creature. At the end of the feast, the newspaper is folded around the empty shells and the bundle is tossed out.

The other way lobster is most commonly eaten is in something called a lobster roll, which is really lobster salad, heavy with mayonnaise, served in a hot dog bun.

In the summers you can eat virtually for free in the Atlantic provinces. All you need is a hoe, some inside information and a fair degree of fortitude. Then the sand beaches, rich with clam beds, are open to you. In the warm months the seashore at low tide is coated with diggers. People also seek quahogs, large soft-shelled mollusks that look like clams. Left whole and steamed like clams, they're about as satisfying as a chunk of B.F. Goodrich, but they are great chopped up, mixed with eggs and bread-crumbs and fried in butter, something like a hamburger. The quahog

31

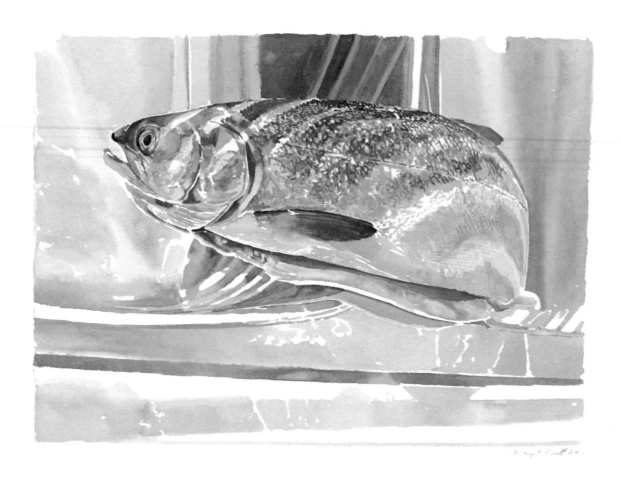

Salmon balanced between two sinks

*When I finished cleaning this fish, it slipped out of
my hands and fell—balanced on the ridge between
the two sinks. It looked as if it were leaping from one
place to another, and banded by light coming
through Venetian blinds, it was too amazing to
ignore. (M.P.)*

burger is found at its best in the Acadian restaurants along the French shore in Nova Scotia. They're also good in chowders, or even battered and deep fried in little pieces.

Mussels, though they have always been very plentiful on the beaches of Nova Scotia, have largely been ignored until quite recently—a baffling oversight. While we in the cities have been paying seven dollars for a bowl of moules marinières, the mussels have been clinging to rocks and lying in shallow waters, there for the taking—unlike clams which require you to dig like a slave for each mouthful. Mussels have other advantages. They are rarely tough, as clams can be, and, carefully gathered, they have little sand, as clams do always.

These two mollusks make up the basis of clambakes, less common in Canada than they are on the eastern seaboard of the United States, but popular none the less. The clams and mussels are gathered, and, if there's time, the clams are left soaking in some seawater with oatmeal or cornmeal in it to coax the animals to spit out the sand trapped in their shells. Then they are scrubbed in seawater. Hot rocks form the bed of the beach fire, then twigs, then layer upon layer of seaweed into which the mollusks are laid. No water is added. They steam by the moisture in the seaweed and within their shells. In fact, many people don't add water to the pot when they steam them at home. They're cooked much the same way you'd cook spinach. Rinse them off, toss them in a pot with a tight-fitting lid and let them cook in their own juices.

Foragers with an eye for the esoteric search out the periwinkles which are easily gathered at low tide. These tiny snails make a wonderful if hard-to-get-at snack. They are often simply boiled in a tin can full of seawater and eaten with a hatpin. Although periwinkles are still much unused, in Toronto the Ho Yuen Chinese restaurant has a dish of periwinkles in black bean and garlic sauce that is one of the best seafood dishes I have ever eaten. The dish probably should be eaten in the bathtub because you have to pick up each tiny winkle with your hands, fish out the meat inside with a toothpick or hat pin, then suck the sauce from the inside and lick it off from the outside. It can take you an hour to eat ten of them.

Sea urchins, very chic in France these days and readily available to anyone with a Swiss bank account, can be gathered along maritime beaches in good years, providing the seagulls don't get them first. The sea urchins are eaten raw, with just a squirt of fresh lemon.

Perhaps as a reaction to the shabby produce often shipped to them from the mainland, Atlantic Canadians are great gatherers of berries and other wild fruits and vegetables—especially wild mushrooms. In the late summer and early fall, the woods and marshes teem with these things. Seasoned mushroom gatherers know their spots and return to them faithfully, year after year. But unlike clam and mussel gatherers, who seem very willing to share their spots, mushroom gatherers are very secretive. "The joy of mushrooms is that once you've found an abundant grouping you can go back to the same spot year after year and harvest an almost priceless crop," said one mushroom picker who wouldn't give an inch when I asked where he gathered his annual bounty. But they needn't be so cautious. Unpractised mushroom seekers are so intimidated by the thought of mushroom poisoning that they wouldn't try an untested spot for love or money. As one gatherer quoted to me on my first foray, "There are old mushroom hunters and bold mushroom hunters, but there are no old, bold mushroom hunters."

I think of food gatherers as a secret sect in Canada. They talk about gathering foods in spiritual and sensual terms. Committed gatherers describe the uplift of getting city hands into country earth, handling fruits warmed by the sun, not chilled by supermarket refrigeration. And gathering the fruits of the earth reminds them of their place on the planet and of their bond with fellow gatherers in other parts of the world. Besides all that, the stuff tastes good and you can get foods you can't find commercially, such as field strawberries or fresh fiddleheads, the tiny first shoots of the ostrich fern. Though recipes can be found that turn them into creamed soup or coat them with Parmesan cheese, they are at their best steamed for only a minute—long enough to take the edge off the crunch—tossed with butter, salt and a couple of grindings of black pepper.

I do my own kind of gathering in the Atlantic provinces. Along well-travelled roads and some not so well travelled are tiny buildings where some of the best food in the provinces can be had. Different from the urban and tourist restaurants, these eateries specialize in fast service of the local specialty, be it clams, scallops or fishburgers. In Newfoundland there's Yummy Good, a road stand that sells fishburgers made with fresh cod. I once spent several days near Covehead in Prince Edward Island because it had a lobster pound on the beach that sold fresh lobster, Malpeque oysters and mackerel at sausage prices. Next door to it a hamburger stand fried them up for a few quarters. I ate them all on the sand, feeling like a millionaire.

These local eateries are the next best thing to home eating. And, as with home eating, you must know someone to find them, though in the past few years, they have increased enormously in number as Atlantic Canadians come to realize how much their real food is appreciated by travellers. When these fried things are good, I don't think there's a better meal to be had. They're sort of eat-with-your-mouth-full, talk-with-your-hands kinds of foods that go well with cold beer and warm friends.

These roadside places are in fact the best places to get indigenous foods. It's here that you'll find the best chowders, made with local fish. You'll find cod's tongues and, if you get there at the right time in the spring, fried salmon in Newfoundland and fried scallops in Digby.

There is something completely satisfying about the freshest of fish dipped in batter and fried quickly in boiling oil so that the fish is soft and the batter is crunchy. I prefer the fish and chips in Newfoundland because cod is usually used there, where haddock or halibut is preferred in Nova Scotia. Cod seems to yield bigger chunks and I find it juicier. If you know where to look in Atlantic Canada, you can have the best fish and chips in the world. I would begin the search on what's locally nicknamed the "chip strip" in St. John's, Newfoundland.

Once along that strip I watched a man eat a huge order of fish and chips. The man sitting at the Arborite counter had been served a platter heaped high with angelically white fresh cod, wrapped in a fragile batter and served with brown chips. Nattily dressed in a herringbone jacket and a plaid bow tie, he methodically pricked the batter of each of the pieces of fish to let the steam escape (a wise idea—you can bite through the batter, which seems innocuous and cool to the tongue and, when it's too late to back out, have a mouthful of steam burns from the fish). He waited for a few minutes to let the steam escape, then he ate the fish reverently, bit by bit, bite by bite, sucking air through his mouth to cool it as he ate.

When he'd eaten the fish, he impaled each fat chip on his fork, one by one, sprinkling it with salt and malt vinegar and biting off the pointed end before swallowing the rest. Toward the end of this repast, which took about half an hour, he called for the strong boiled tea so popular in Newfoundland. When he had finally finished, he dabbed the corners of his mouth with the paper napkin, dusted off his knees, paid the bill and left. The extraordinary fish and chips had been dispatched with the respect that was their due.

There are many such meals to be found throughout the Atlantic provinces. On the Bay of Fundy in Nova Scotia, there are countless little stands selling deep-fried scallops. These little nuggets, crisp and hot on the outside yielding to a soft, juicy centre inside, are alone worth the trip. The aptly named World's Best Clams on the south shore across the bay matches the scallops with clams. There are other clam stands as good, but I like World's Best also for their world's best fish fritters, which I feel particularly qualified to mention since I think I have sampled more of them than almost anyone else I know. There's also McLeod's Canteen in

Green Bay on the way to World's Best, which has the best chips in the region and the best chowders and the best pies.

The best eateries in Atlantic Canada really are the restaurants that cook the local stuff the same way it's cooked in homes. And when they cook it the way they do in homes, they serve it the same way—with lots of breads and sweet baked goods.

Baked goods are prominent in home-cooked Atlantic meals, and often they are served at the beginning of the meal as well as throughout. This custom is probably a holdover from the days before central heating, when the stove was also used to keep the kitchen warm. The family lived mostly in the kitchen in winter, huddled near the big iron stove which usually had soup simmering on top and cakes and breads rising within. Fuel was expensive, and efforts were made to conserve it, mainly by limiting the heating to one room. In older houses, nearly every room in the house can be closed off from the other, so that the traditional Atlantic home has more doors than windows. The windows that there are tend to face the road, away from the sea which, while it's very picturesque, blows fierce winds. Visitors to these provinces often comment on the large picture windows facing the road and ignoring the sea. Maybe it's also because it's more fun to watch who's driving by on the road.

Like many Atlantic Canadians, Winnie Allen of Pleasant River, Nova Scotia, spends an average of five hours a day at her wood stove baking brown breads and pies. "I pile the pies high with apples," she says. "I hate those skimpy pies with no filling." She bakes for bake sales, too, so her fame has spread throughout the community.

A sampling of the better bake sales might bring molasses cookies, molasses cakes (called lassy cake in Newfoundland) and potato fudge (grated potatoes instead of flour makes for creamy candy). If the sale is in the summer, the berry pies are stunning. If it's in the winter when there's less produce but more time to decorate, the love of handicrafts becomes evident. At a community sale in Beach Meadows, Nova Scotia, I was fascinated by a cake constructed to the exact specifications of a Rubik's cube, which, as they say, would have been a sin to eat.

Whether you're eating a meal at home or along the way, you must watch your intake. The servings in Atlantic Canada are enormous. The problem with these restaurants, many of which are off the beaten track, is that there's nowhere to walk off the meal. You just get back in your car and bump along the highway for another hour or so until your distended stomach settles somewhere to the south of your collarbone.

One of the best places in Atlantic Canada to get a feeling for the largesse of the home cooking is at York's Dining Room in Perth-Andover in northern New Brunswick near the Maine border. But it is quite a bit off the beaten track. If you are travelling east from Quebec, you have to detour to go there. The roadway at six p.m. early in the week was filled with cars bearing American license plates. It is one of those Canadian treasures that they know about and we don't. Barely seconds after you have ordered your meal, your table top is covered with tea biscuits and fresh butter, with crisply deep-fried corn fritters afloat in maple syrup (I find it impossible to exercise any restraint when it comes to fritters of any kind, and had eaten three of these before the meal came). As well there is banana bread, raisin bread, coleslaw and pickles. There were two of us at our huge table, so to go with all the breads, the waitress brought two huge bowls of butter.

This kind of home cooking can also be found in the inns and bed-and-breakfast places throughout Atlantic Canada. Though the bed-and-breakfast concept is becoming more popular in other parts of the country, in the Atlantic Provinces it has a longer tradition. They're more like the family-run guest house/bed-and-breakfast places found in England and in New England in the United States.

The Marshlands Inn in New Brunswick, near Mount Allison University, is probably the best known. Countless articles have attested to the perfect prettiness of this sprawling white house with its cared-for country-inn furnishings which include four-poster beds and footed bathtubs, little letter desks and open fireplaces. But what is really appealing is its dining room, which for the many years of its operation has served local home-style food.

On my last visit I had wild mushrooms which had been picked that morning from the nearby Tantramar marshes and served on buttered homemade bread. At the Marshlands, as at the York Dining Room, you are immediately faced with baked goods which are difficult to resist on an empty stomach. On other occasions I've had fresh salmon topped with creamy white egg sauce, roast beef with Yorkshire pudding, lobster salads, fish n' brewis and cod au gratin. But it's the desserts that help make it so special—snow pudding, light and airy, with an eggy custard sauce; homemade berry pies served with hard sauce; stewed foxberries and, in season, real strawberry shortcake and fresh strawberry ice cream.

The smaller inns throughout the Atlantic provinces must be more diligently sought because they are not well advertised. Travellers pass around informational tidbits and one can only hope you hear about the best places before you go, rather than after you get home. I've often settled for stale white rolls and Tang for breakfast, only to learn that half a mile down the road was a sumptuous meal fit for a queen.

One such breakfast included a huge frying pan filled with a wonderful French toast, made fresh as each bleary-eyed guest arrived. Our hostess had used thick slices of French bread that she had soaked in beaten eggs, milk, vanilla and a shot of undiluted orange juice. They were served with maple syrup, fresh raspberries and peaches, since that was the season for those fruits, but they could as easily have been served with chopped orange or cooked apples or even sliced bananas. She said the secret of the best French toast is to soak the bread in the egg mixture before it is fried in butter. The long soaking infuses the bread with egg and by the time it has been cooked, it's like eating long slabs of a delicious custard, fried in butter and awash in maple syrup.

This particular breakfast in New Brunswick also included fresh home-made muffins, pans full of bacon and sausage, juice and coffee. The room and breakfast for two was about thirty dollars, which seemed to me to be a pretty good deal. And, after a while it's even okay to face breakfast with strangers. Everyone exchanges bed and breakfast experiences, so you wind up with some good stories and a terrific list of other places. There's one in Cape Breton that serves fresh fish for breakfast, didn't you know, or another where you can have fresh lamb or yet another in Newfoundland that serves fish n' brewis on Saturday nights. You must treasure these exchanges over the breakfast tables. It's the only way for a traveller, who doesn't have an Aunt Mary in Atlantic Canada, to have home cooking.

The real culinary wealth of Atlantic Canada exists on platters heaped in home kitchens and served at private dining tables. It exists in tiny taverns, church bake sales and roadside eateries that are few and far between and known best by local residents who seldom go out to eat. To eat well in Atlantic Canada it helps to know someone like Winnie Allen of Pleasant River, or someone who can take you to the church bake sales at Broad Cove, where a couple of years ago they took out an ad in the paper to apologize for running out of food. Then you can join the locals to dine wonderfully on the produce of backyard gardens, on the extraordinary bounty of fish and game and on the baked goods produced in their kitchens.

The food Atlantic ex-patriots describe with longing is there—just as wonderful as they said it was. But it's hiding. It's hiding in the home kitchens and cowering in church basements. It has written a Dear John letter to the West and stayed home with mother.

Maybe soon they'll bring it out and let the rest of us have a taste. They needn't worry. Their secret is safe with us.

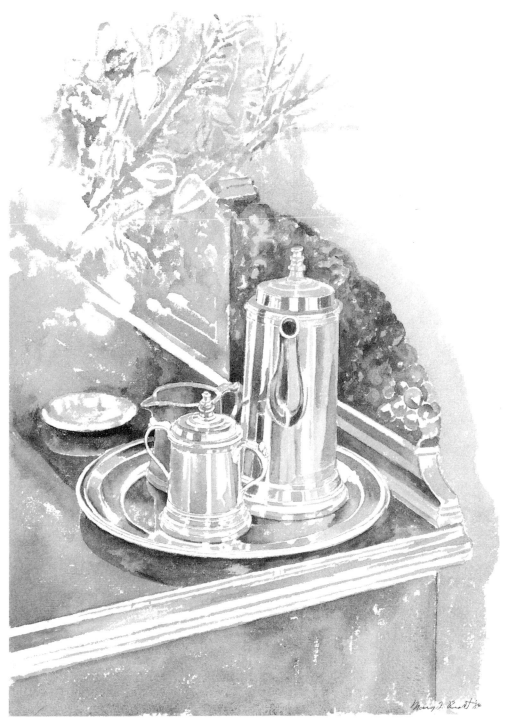

Pewter tea things

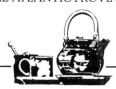

SEAFOOD CHOWDER

A traditional Atlantic chowder is made with fish or shellfish, canned milk, potatoes, onions and is served with a dollop of butter. This version, which comes from a Nova Scotia fisherman and uses sour cream, fresh cream and thyme, is quite different and very good.

When reheating leftover chowder, it may be necessary to add a little more milk or cream, because the fish and potatoes will have absorbed some of the liquid.

1	medium onion, minced	1
1 Tbsp	butter	15 mL
1 1/2 tsp	thyme	7 mL
1 1/4 tsp	celery salt	6 mL
2 cups	whipping cream	500 mL
8 oz	haddock or halibut fillets	250 g
6 oz	scallops, chopped	150 g
3 oz	lobster meat, cooked and chopped	75 g
3/4 cup	sour cream	175 mL
3	medium potatoes, peeled, cooked and diced	3
1 1/4 cups	milk	300 mL
1 tsp	salt	5 mL
1/2 tsp	freshly ground pepper	2 mL
	Paprika for garnish	

1. Cook the onion in the butter until transparent. Add the thyme and celery salt. Remove from heat.

2. In a saucepan, pour the whipping cream over the fish fillets. Cover, bring to a boil and simmer slowly for 10 minutes, or until the fish flakes easily. Remove the fish with a slotted spoon, then break into small pieces and remove any bones.

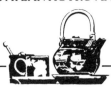

3. Add the onion mixture and the scallops to the poaching liquid. Bring barely to a boil, then simmer for about 1 minute, or until the scallops are opaque. If the chowder is not to be eaten immediately, refrigerate everything at this stage.

4. Just before serving, add the fish, lobster, sour cream, potatoes and milk. Heat through, but do not allow to boil. Season with salt and pepper.

5. Ladle into soup bowls. Sprinkle with paprika. Serve immediately.

Serves 4 to 6

—The Zwicker Inn, Mahone Bay, Nova Scotia

RABBIT IN FIFTEEN GARLIC CLOVES

Do not be intimidated by the large amount of garlic in this recipe. Slowly simmered, it becomes sweet and delicious. This dish is based on an Acadian recipe from New Brunswick. Serve the rabbit with white rice or plain boiled potatoes.

1	rabbit, cut in pieces	1
2 Tbsp	olive oil	25 mL
1 tsp	salt	5 mL
1/2 tsp	freshly ground pepper	2 mL
15	cloves garlic, peeled and left whole	15
1/2 cup	water	125 mL
	Parsley, several sprigs for garnish	

1. In a heavy frying pan, cook the rabbit pieces in the olive oil until well browned on all sides.

2. Add the salt, pepper and garlic cloves and cook for a few minutes.

3. Add the water. Cover the pan and simmer for 2 hours, or until the rabbit is tender, checking occasionally to make sure that the liquid has not evaporated.

4. Serve and garnish with parsley.

Serves 4

—La Fine Grobe, Nigadoo, New Brunswick

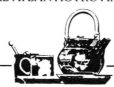

FETOYA

These yeast buns stuffed with fresh spinach or chard were brought to the Atlantic provinces by Lebanese immigrants. Flavoured with allspice, lemon juice and fresh mint, they are among the best foods I have ever eaten. You can make your own bread dough for the casing, though the supermarket frozen variety works fine in this recipe. Don't be alarmed at the amount of spinach or chard—it cooks down to the appropriate amount.

3 lb	white bread dough, thawed	1.5 kg
18 cups	fresh spinach or Swiss chard, or 3 10-oz/284-g packages	4.5 L
2	medium onions, coarsely chopped	2
1/3 cup	fresh lemon juice	75 mL
1 1/2 cups	corn oil	375 mL
2 tsp	salt	10 mL
1/2 tsp	freshly ground pepper	2 mL
1 tsp	ground allspice	5 mL
1 cup	fresh mint leaves, or 1/2 cup/125 mL dried	250 mL

1. Place the bread dough in an oiled bowl. Oil the top of the dough, cover and let rise in a warm place until doubled in bulk, about 1 1/2 hours. Punch down and allow to swell slightly. Punch down and divide equally into 15 pieces.

2. While the dough is rising, rinse and trim the spinach. Cut into bite-sized pieces.

3. Combine the spinach, onions, lemon juice, corn oil, salt, pepper, allspice and mint. Mix thoroughly.

4. To assemble the buns, roll each piece of dough on a lightly floured surface into a circle about 8 in/20 cm in diameter. Trim roughly to a triangular shape.

5. Place approximately 3/4 cup/175 mL spinach mixture in the centre of each triangle. Fold over the edges and pinch to seal edges and corners. Press buns with the palm of your hand to flatten slightly.

6. Preheat oven to 375°F/190°C.

7. Rub the buns on both sides with a little flour. Brush lightly with oil and place on a well-oiled baking sheet. Snip a few vents in the top of each bun with scissors or a knife.

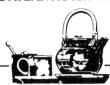

8. Bake in 3 batches on the lowest rack of the oven for 5 to 6 minutes. Turn the buns over and continue baking for 5 to 6 minutes, or until golden brown. Serve warm or at room temperature with yogurt.

Makes 15 buns

—*Margaret Sapp, Liverpool, Nova Scotia*

COD AU GRATIN

Cod baked in a cheese sauce is a very popular dish in Newfoundland. It is also very good. The dish may be made with fresh or salted cod. If salt cod is used, the fish must be freshened first by soaking it for at least twelve hours, changing the water once or twice during that time.

1 lb	cod fillets	500 g
¼ cup	butter	50 mL
¼ cup	flour	50 mL
2 cups	milk	500 mL
½ cup	grated Cheddar cheese	125 mL
½ tsp	salt	2 mL
½ tsp	freshly ground pepper	2 mL

1. Preheat oven to 425°F/220°C.

2. Cover the cod fillets with water. Bring to a boil and cook for 8 to 10 minutes, or just until the cod begins to flake at the touch of a fork.

3. Meanwhile, prepare the white sauce by melting the butter in a large saucepan. When it begins to bubble, add the flour. Blend well and cook for several minutes but do not brown.

4. Slowly stir in the milk. Continue cooking the sauce, stirring constantly, until it begins to thicken.

5. Mix in half the cheese. Add salt and pepper. (If you have used salt cod, additional salt will probably not be necessary.)

6. Break the cod into large chunks and arrange in a buttered casserole. Pour the cheese sauce over the fish. Sprinkle the remaining cheese over the top.

7. Bake for 10 minutes, or just until the fish is heated through and the top is nicely browned.

Serves 4

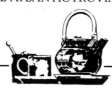

TEA GOOSE

This is the best recipe for goose that I have ever tried. The tea marinade helps coax all of the excess fat out of the goose and at the same time it tenderizes the meat and lets it absorb the flavours of the herbs and wine.

1	8-lb/4-kg goose, fresh or thawed	1
2 Tbsp	white vinegar	25 mL
	Marinade:	
1	onion, chopped	1
1	carrot, chopped	1
1	stalk celery, chopped	1
4	cloves garlic, peeled and lightly crushed	4
1 tsp	thyme	5 mL
1	bay leaf	1
2 Tbsp	chopped parsley	25 mL
4	whole cloves	4
1 tsp	rosemary	5 mL
1 tsp	basil	5 mL
½ tsp	marjoram	2 mL
½ tsp	nutmeg	2 mL
½ tsp	cinnamon	2 mL
2 Tbsp	vegetable oil	25 mL
¼ cup	red or white wine vinegar	50 mL
1 cup	red or white wine	250 mL
½ cup	gin	125 mL
4 to 6 cups	strong tea	1 to 1.5L

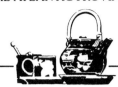

1. Remove the excess pouches of fat from the goose. Wipe the goose inside and out with the white vinegar.

2. Combine all the ingredients for the marinade.

3. Put the goose and the marinade in a clean, strong plastic bag. Press out the air and tie the bag securely. Leave in a cool place for 24 hours, occasionally turning the bag and massaging the marinade into the meat.

4. Preheat oven to 350°F/180°C.

5. Discard the marinade and salt and pepper the goose inside and out. Roast for 1 hour. Remove goose from the oven and, with a fork, prick it around the legs and wings to allow fat to escape.

6. Cover the goose with foil. Continue roasting for 3 hours.

7. Uncover the goose and roast for another 30 minutes, or until the breast meat is tender to a fork. Let stand 15 minutes before carving to allow the juices to settle back in the meat.

Serves 4 to 6

—*Trudi Clements, Liverpool, Nova Scotia*

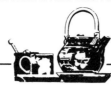

LOBSTER WITH TOMATOES

The freshest of lobster makes this dish special; cooking with lobster that has not been pre-cooked makes an astounding difference. Also, the shells lend flavour. If you buy the live lobsters in a city market, don't try to preserve them in the bathtub—they need seawater, not fluoride. They should survive overnight in a cool place, but once they have been killed, they must be used immediately.

1	2-lb/1-kg lobster, freshly killed but not cooked	1
1	large onion, finely chopped	1
2	cloves garlic, finely chopped	2
2 Tbsp	olive oil	25 mL
1/4 cup	brandy	50 mL
2	tomatoes, peeled and quartered	2
1 tsp	tomato paste	5 mL
1 tsp	granulated sugar	5 mL
1/2 tsp	salt	2 mL
1/2 tsp	freshly ground pepper	2 mL

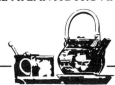

1. Kill the lobster by inserting a knife at the base of the head. The butcher may do this for you if you prefer, but the lobster must be used immediately.

2. Cook the onion and garlic in the olive oil until soft.

3. With a sharp knife or cleaver, chop the lobster *in the shell* crosswise in 1-in/2.5-cm chunks along the length of the tail and body.

4. Remove the green sac at the base of the brain and discard. Reserve the red coral (roe) if there is any and the greenish tomalley (liver).

5. Cook the lobster pieces with the onion and garlic until the lobster shell turns red. It is important that the shell be a definite red, or the meat will be hard to remove. Still, be careful not to overcook. Once the shell is red, reduce the heat immediately.

6. When the heat has been reduced, pour in the brandy. Let it heat for a moment, then ignite it with a match. The flame will go out as soon as the alcohol has been burned off.

7. Remove the lobster from the pan. Remove the meat from the shell and reserve both.

8. Return the shell to the pan. Add the tomatoes, tomato paste, sugar, salt and pepper. Boil the mixture gently until it becomes quite thick.

9. Remove all the shell pieces from the pan and discard.

10. Return the meat, including the coral and tomalley, to the pan and simmer in the sauce for 5 minutes. Serve immediately with buttered rice.

Serves 2

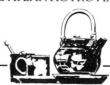

COD JIGGER'S DINNER

This fisherman's meal of salt beef, vegetables and pease porridge is part of a traditional Newfoundland dinner. Pease porridge, the soothing stuff of nursery rhymes, is an old English and Irish dish made by boiling split yellow peas in a cloth bag until they are soft. The Newfoundland pease porridge gains extra flavour from the salt beef and vegetables. Once the dish is cooked, it is important to remove the meat, vegetables and peas from the pot while the water is still boiling, to prevent the fat from settling on the food.

4 lb	salt beef or corned beef	2 kg
8 oz	split yellow peas	250 g
6	potatoes, peeled and quartered	6
6	carrots, scraped and cut in half lengthwise	6
1	turnip, peeled and cut into 8 wedges	1
1	head cabbage, cut in wedges	1
1/4 cup	butter	50 mL
	Salt and freshly ground pepper to taste	

1. If you are using salt beef, soak it overnight in cold water. Cut the meat into 2-in/5-cm pieces and remove excess fat.

2. Place the meat in a large soup pot and cover completely with water. Put the peas in a sturdy cotton bag or several layers of cheesecloth tied securely into a bag. Suspend the bag in the water by hooking or tying the tied end onto the handle of the soup pot. Boil the meat and the peas for 2½ hours.

3. Add the potatoes, carrots and turnip. Cook for 15 minutes.

4. Add the cabbage and cook for 10 minutes more. Do not overcook or the cabbage will become too soft.

5. While the cabbage is cooking, remove the peas from the water and turn them into a heated bowl. Mash them with butter and season with salt and pepper.

6. Remove the vegetables and meat from the pot while the water is still boiling. Drain and chop the cabbage.

7. Arrange the meat on a serving platter surrounded by the vegetables and pease porridge. Mustard pickles or pickled beets make tasty condiments.

Serves 6

—Mary Darcy, St. John's, Newfoundland

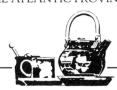

PLEASANT RIVER BAKED BEANS

Winnie Allen of Pleasant River, Nova Scotia, is famous for her baked beans because they are unusually rich and flavourful. Serve them with brown bread, sausages and a glass of ale. In Quebec, baked beans are sometimes served for breakfast with fried eggs and sliced ripe tomatoes.

2 lb	dried beans (yellow-eyed or navy)	1 kg
1 tsp	dry mustard	5 mL
1 tsp	salt	5 mL
1/4 tsp	freshly ground pepper	1 mL
1	medium onion, sliced	1
1/4 cup	brown sugar	50 mL
1/2 cup	molasses	125 mL
1/2 cup	ketchup	125 mL
8 oz	bacon ends or slices	250 g
8 oz	salt pork	250 g

1. In a large pot, cover the beans with cold water, bring to a boil and simmer for 2 minutes. Remove from heat and let stand, tightly covered, for 1 hour.

2. Make sure the beans are still fully covered in water and then bring them to a boil again. Reduce heat and simmer for about 1 more hour, or until the skins burst when you take a few beans on a spoon and blow on them.

3. Preheat oven to 250°F/120°C.

4. Drain the beans, reserving the cooking water. Place the beans in a large covered crock or casserole.

5. Combine the mustard, salt, pepper, onion, brown sugar, molasses and ketchup with 1 cup/250 mL of the reserved cooking water. Pour over the beans. Add more water if necessary to cover.

6. Stir in the bacon.

7. Cover the salt pork with boiling water and let stand for 2 minutes. Drain and cut gashes 1 in/2.5 cm deep every 1/2 in/1 cm along the length of the meat, without cutting through the rind. Push the salt pork down into the beans until all but the rind is covered.

8. Cover the crock and bake for 6 to 8 hours, or until the beans are tender. During the cooking add boiling water if necessary to keep the beans covered. Uncover beans for the last hour of baking so the rind will brown.

Serves 10 to 12

—*Winnie Allen, Pleasant River, Nova Scotia*

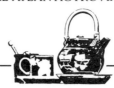

APPLE CAKE WITH CIDER GLAZE

The Annapolis Valley in Nova Scotia is well known for its apples, and in the fall you can find varieties that are no longer commercially available. Nova Scotia apple cider is very good, too, especially if you can find your way past the commercial bottled stuff and into the barns where it is fermented slow and strong.

1½ cups	vegetable oil	375 mL
2 cups	granulated sugar	500 mL
3	eggs	3
2 tsp	vanilla	10 mL
3 cups	all-purpose flour	750 mL
1 tsp	baking soda	5 mL
2 tsp	cinnamon	10 mL
1 tsp	freshly grated nutmeg	5 mL
½ tsp	salt	2 mL
3 cups	unpeeled and diced tart apples (such as Cortland or Northern Spy)	750 mL
1 cup	walnut pieces	250 mL
	Glaze:	
¼ cup	butter	50 mL
¼ cup	brown sugar	50 mL
¼ cup	granulated sugar	50 mL
¼ cup	apple cider	50 mL

1. Preheat oven to 325°F/160°C.

2. Combine the oil and sugar. Beat in the eggs, one at a time. Stir in the vanilla.

3. Sift together the flour, baking soda, cinnamon, nutmeg and salt. Add to the oil mixture and combine thoroughly.

4. Add the diced apples and walnuts and mix well.

5. Pour the batter into a buttered and floured Bundt pan. Bake for 1¼ hours or until a skewer inserted into the centre of the cake comes out clean. Remove the cake from the oven and let it sit for 10 minutes. Invert onto a platter.

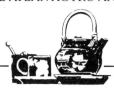

6. To prepare the glaze, combine the butter, sugars and cider in a saucepan. Boil for 1 or 2 minutes. Remove from heat and brush over warm cake.

Serves 10 to 12

—Kathy Chute, Milton, Nova Scotia

COTTAGE PUDDING WITH MOLASSES SAUCE

This is one of those desserts that you find in people's homes in Atlantic Canada and are somehow never as good when you eat them in restaurants.

1¾ cups	all-purpose flour	425 mL
2 tsp	baking powder	10 mL
½ tsp	salt	2 mL
¼ cup	butter, at room temperature	50 mL
¾ cup	granulated sugar	175 mL
1	large egg	1
1 tsp	vanilla	5 mL
¾ cup	milk	175 mL
	Molasses Sauce:	
1 cup	molasses	250 mL
2 Tbsp	butter	25 mL

1. Preheat oven to 350°F/180°C.
2. Blend together the flour, baking powder and salt.
3. In a large bowl, cream the butter and sugar together until light. Add the egg and beat in thoroughly.
4. In a separate bowl, blend together the vanilla and milk.
5. Add the dry ingredients to the creamed mixture alternately with the milk. Blend until smooth.
6. Pour batter into a buttered and floured 9-in/2.5-L square pan. Bake for 30 minutes or until the pudding is golden on top and springs back when touched in the middle.
7. Combine the molasses and butter and heat slowly. Do not boil. Cut the cottage pudding into squares and serve warm with the hot molasses sauce.

Serves 6

—Mary Darcy, St. John's, Newfoundland

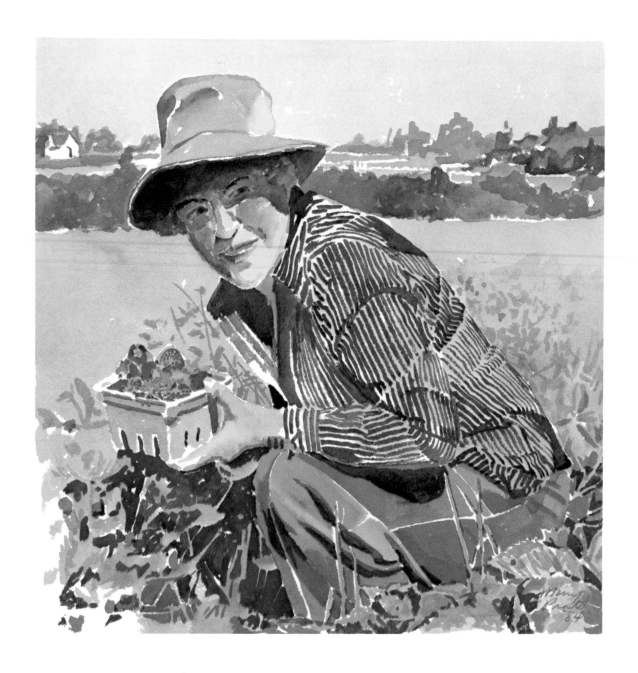

Katherine picking strawberries

*My mother used to pick enough strawberries for all
her jam and jelly, and have lots left over for dipping
into the sugar bowl. She is a very pretty lady, but
never prettier than when she's in a garden. (M.P.)*

QUEBEC

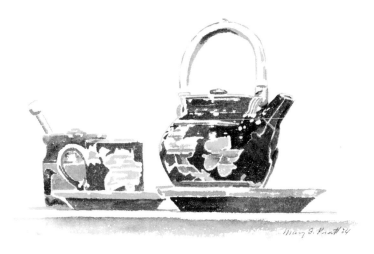

Quebec is the culinary capital of Canada. Its traditional foods have defined Canadian cuisine for other nations (even if the rest of the world didn't know much about Canadian food, it knew Oka cheese and maple syrup), and its modern chefs describe a standard for other provinces. Quebec is the home of more food societies than any other province and, perhaps as a consequence, the location of a hefty number of weight-reducing enterprises.

As I travelled across Canada, I saved Quebec as my reward for all the foods I hadn't liked in other provinces. When I ate whale blubber in the North and dulse in New Brunswick, I promised myself I'd make up for it in Quebec. Once I got there, there wasn't anything I would miss. I wanted to eat everything—and did. In a Westmount living room in Montreal, a Chinese chef cooked me a six-course dinner of kosher Chinese food. I spent an afternoon on a private railway car that had been converted into a travelling dining room and ate one of the poshest meals ever. And once, to repair from the excesses of eating that I had done on a two-week toot, I checked into a convent for Gregorian chants and poached eggs on toast.

Quebeckers acknowledge their good food. In most other provinces, if you ask local residents what the best thing to eat is, they will send you to someone who does Cordon Bleu cookery; in Quebec they will send you to their neighbour who makes the world's best tourtière.

More than in any other province, Quebec's government concerns itself with its cuisine. There, eating well is a matter of official policy. The government goes to great lengths to catalogue and describe what people eat and how it relates to what they used to eat. The government is also anxious to direct how people will be eating in the future. In 1984, the centre of technological research of the Quebec institute of tourism sponsored a series of pamphlets on the regional cuisine of Quebec, describing eighteen regions, each with its own specialties and cooking techniques.

The recipes of today's Quebec are sophisticated and light, in keeping with the modern climate of using fresh produce and manipulating it no more than is necessary to provide a setting for the natural flavours. These contemporary dishes are a far cry from the heavy, long-cooked foods we associate with rural Quebec. Fresh trout is sautéed only lightly and served with a sauce of watercress; Quebec's famous Brome Lake duck is cooked pink in the centre, as required by forward-looking chefs, flavoured only with grains of freshly ground white and black peppercorns, and accompanied with hazelnuts corrupted only by a hint of ground almonds. Rabbit, that old Quebec standby, no longer cowers in pies and stews. In the new Quebec it is cooked in Cognac with honey and shallots; or it is flamed with Calvabec (Quebec's answer to Calvados brandy) and served with beans. But these beans aren't baked for days in slow ovens and baptized with maple syrup. Quebec's new beans are puréed with cream and laid gently alongside the rabbit, the meal napped with a sauce of liver, shallots and garlic. They're not quaint or hearty; they're smooth and almost, well, delicate.

Delicate is not a word that might have been used to describe the traditional cuisine of Quebec. Beans baked for hours in brick ovens, embalmed in maple syrup and eaten with bread and salt pork. Or pea soup made with dried peas simmered with salt pork or fat bacon, bubbled at the back of the stove long enough to moisten the peas—and heat the kitchen. Or cipaille and its more famous cousin, tourtière.

The two meat pies are the dishes into which all the gastronomic philosophy of pioneer Quebec is baked. The pies are the best examples of how to get the most calories in the form of protein, starch and fat into the smallest reasonable space. The dishes were designed to provide the caloric whomp that was needed by people working from daylight to dusk in cold places. They built log cabins and fortresses in the bitter cold, and while no one has estimated exactly how many calories it takes to build a stockade, it is not likely it could be accomplished on kiwi.

Like the pioneers of other Canadian provinces, Quebec's settlers were of peasant stock, not from the nobility who could afford to develop tastes for daintier meals with ingredients and spices that had to be brought from far away. For the pioneers, meats were gravied and encased in pastry. Breads were sliced thick and crusty and reinforced with spreadings of hot salt pork if the bread was part of the main meal, or covered in maple syrup and thick cream if it was dessert.

Some of these early Quebec dishes were as daunting to prepare as they were to digest. The cipaille (pronounced sea-pie and thought to be derived either from six-pâtés or from the English sea pie which was made with fish) is three layers of pastry which enclose various types of game and gravies. The recipe I have for cipaille presumes that my husband has just returned from the hunt. It begins with the instruction "Bone rabbits and chicken." That done, I would mix the meat with some onions and lay them in the fat from rendered salt pork. Then I would weave the pie: a layer of pastry on the bottom, a layer of meat and fat on top, then another layer of pastry, another of meat, and then a finishing blanket of pastry.

The secret to cipaille is the middle layer of pastry, which is a quilt's worth of little squares laid side by side, so that the centre layer can expand in the heat. The middle layer of Quebec cipaille operates on the same principle as Canadian sidewalks. They are laid not in long cement strips that will crack and contract from the effects of the freezing winters and hot summers, but in squares with cracks in between to allow for expansion. I once tried to make cipaille using three solid sheets of pastry. The pastry in the middle herniated in the baking, allowing my rabbit layer to bulge into my chicken layer. After the pie was cooked, the middle layer was flexible and wet and the outer layer impervious to a sharp fork, providing a kind of bastille for the layers of meat inside, which were tough and raw.

Tourtière is the more famous Quebec meat pie, so famous that along with pea soup, it has become the cliché of Québecois cuisine, often served when Canadian specialties are expected. Its principles are generally the same as for the cipaille, but there are only two layers of pastry and the meat (traditionally pork) is ground up. A less commonly known style from the Lac St. Jean region is filled with cubed meat and potatoes. There are a million different versions of the ground-meat style in Quebec, and even a few outside the province, including a hand-held tourtière turnover designed for an international convention of cooking school teachers who met in Toronto, and by a meat company in Kitchener, Ontario, that sells it frozen in packages. The package states that tourtière was a favourite meal of the habitants and usually served as the main course at the reveillon feast on New Year's Eve. It also promises that tourtière is truly a Canadian dish, which must come as a great relief to the Quebeckers who have been giving the stuff to their kids since the seventeenth century.

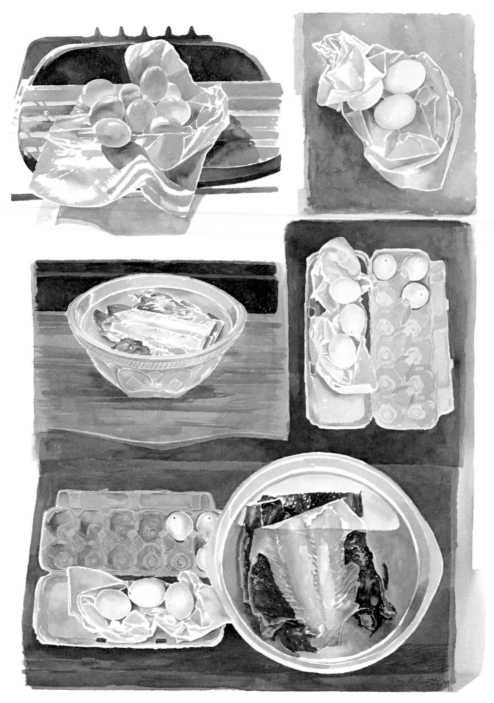

Five images of Good Friday

*Blown eggs sit like bubbles on a crumpled paper
towel. Light pours over and through them, so
translucent and so perfect. (M.P.)*

In fact, Quebec has one of the longest histories of all the provinces and, at least by reputation, is the province with the longest history of a concern for food. French settlers brought with them their preoccupation with what was on their tables from their mother country, adapting the produce they found in Canada to their natives dishes. It is not surprising that Canada's first gourmet club was established by a Frenchman, Samuel de Champlain, in 1604 in Nova Scotia, four years before he founded Quebec City, to distract his men from the hardships of the new country.

The French in Canada have a long history as an identifiable and cohesive group and in that way Quebec differs from western Canada whose population is made up of many different groups with varied approaches to the local foodstuffs. The celebration of food in Quebec is a tangible part of the culture. In nearly every festivity, including those not necessarily food-related, like New Year's Eve, food plays a major part.

Anyone wishing exposure to the traditional foods of rural Quebec need only find their way to one of the province's many sugar shacks that provide the paying public with an afternoon's festivities and education into the food life of the habitants. At the sugar shacks, maple sap is gathered, converted into maple syrup and employed in nearly every dish imaginable. Don't, however, do as I did and visit one in the heat of a June afternoon. On that steamy day I ate eggs poached in maple syrup, ham with maple syrup used as a sauce, soufflé with maple syrup poured over it, maple sugar candies, maple syrup cake and maple syrup cookies. I brought home with me some maple sugar candy which I grated on top of a dish of bananas and yoghurt. It was the best yet, probably because the tartness of the yoghurt interfered with the sweetness of the candy.

On a better-advised visit in January, I had maple syrup the plainest way you can have it, which is simply trailed through the snow until it becomes like industrial-strength gold taffy with enough integrity to dismantle your bridgework. I have mixed feelings about maple syrup on eggs, unless the eggs are first welded to bread and turned into French toast, despite a friend's promise that eggs fried in butter and a bit of maple syrup would make me about as happy as I'm likely to get. But I do feel that whoever conceived of the marriage of maple syrup to smoked ham was inspired.

Quebeckers' love of sweetness is legendary. (The joke about the most popular breakfast being Pepsi and Mae West—a large chocolate cookie filled with cream—is not a complete fabrication.) Even in these days of sugar consciousness, Quebeckers still view the sugar-free soft drinks with suspicion. Quebec, in fact, has one of the highest rates of dental cavities in the civilized world, an honour attributable in no small way to the lust for sweet.

A couple of years ago, I was one of the judges at a strawberry pie contest on Ile d'Orléans, a lush little island in the St. Lawrence near Quebec City. The contest was part of that area's annual strawberry festival, organized in celebration of their stunning crop of berries—both the large cultivated strawberries we find in supermarkets, and the tiny field berries with their intense crimson flavour. These luscious fruits are the descendants of the original wild strawberry, found in abundance by Canada's earliest settlers. The crops on Ile d'Orléans are especially delicious. During the short picking season in early July, the fields are crowded with the backsides of islanders and visitors filling baskets and pails to heaping.

The rules of the contest required that all entries be variations on a strawberry pie. The limits were stretched. A large brioche was filled with fresh berries and surrounded by piles of whipped cream. In another, strawberries were set in oversized meringue puffs, each large enough to sleep a newborn baby.

One bizarre entry was more a cake than a pie. The huge square was decorated like the American flag with strawberries and dots of blueberries to designate the stars and stripes. There were also many traditional two-crust pies, but with air vents in every conceivable shape. One glorious entry offered a large, highly decorated open-faced tart surrounded by several similar tarts. "Like a queen and her handmaidens," whispered a wide-eyed admirer to her friend.

No matter how unique the variations, these pies all had one thing in common. They were very, very sweet. By the time I was at pie three in the tasting I knew I'd had enough. By pie five I was satisfied beyond any childish appetite; pie eight and my ears were ringing; pie eleven and I began to consider the back exit. But I stayed through pie fourteen and even tasted the American flag, perhaps because of pressure from the local judges, who thought it was awfully nice.

They in the main were responsible for awarding first prize to the fluted pie shell piped with sweet cream and filled with red Jello into which whole berries had been gracefully set.

I don't want to leave you with the impression that I'm above this sort of caloric excess. I'd give up my stove for just one plateful of warm bread, soaked with fresh cream and dripping with maple syrup. And that goes in spades for salt pork. When salt pork has just been pulled from a pot where it has been flavouring boiling vegetables and chicken, hot and steamy, it almost spreads like pâté. If you can imagine the flavour of hot, salty-smoky fat on warm bread, slightly flavoured with maple syrup, you'll have some idea of why the habitants were so glad to come in from the cold.

I learned about the wonderfulness of salt pork one overstuffed afternoon at the table of Quebec's ambassadress of the kitchen, Mme Benoit. She is the doyenne of Canadian food writers, a television personality and the best known of public cooks who has parlayed an interest in food into a lifetime career and an enterprise that includes many cookbooks and a string of kitchenware shops.

Mme Benoit and her husband live near Sutton in the Eastern Townships, in a farmhouse filled with Canadian antiques and the kind of ambience that comes from years of living in and loving a home. Much of the house is taken over by the huge kitchen, pantry and dining room that would be the envy of any serious gourmand or cook.

Our lunch was laid out on the table in the sunny dining room, and the name of each dish was described on a pretty ribboned place card sitting in front of it: meat loaf ringed with bacon, rolled with sausages and served with grainy buckwheat pilaf, plus a thick and warming vegetable soup. And those were just starters.

The main course was a whole chicken, boiled with vegetables and a huge chunk of salt pork. With it she served three types of bread from a local bakery, each completely sliced, then reformed and held together with a length of ribbon. Until Mme Benoit laid a chunk of salt pork on my plate and handed me a piece of bread to spread it on, I had assumed it was in the pot to give flavour to the chicken and vegetables. I was horrified at the thought of what even one bite of that dripping fat might add to me. I took a bite, finished that slice and had another. It was wonderful.

I have always been curious about the home kitchens of professional cooks and was no less so at Mme Benoit's, despite the enormous lunch that had left me close to comatose. There is nothing that can make you more cynical about professional cooks and food writers than opening their fridge doors. The insides of some of these famous ice-boxes could disillusion a saint: ketchup bottles, hard, spotty cheeses, green pizza and limp vegetables. Behind cupboard doors, commercial canned goods and packaged mixes line the shelves of some of Canada's most fastidious proponents of natural foods. Not at Mme Benoit's. Each of her two refrigerators was filled with the most laudable of edibles: homemade condiments in shiny jars, carefully wrapped fresh cheeses, tightly sealed fresh vegetables, homemade rose vinegar and homemade yoghurt. The only commercial product was a jar of Syrian pickled mushrooms.

Open shelves on the walls were lined with wine bottles and rows of jars of dried legumes and homemade preserves. Whatever wall space that was left was taken up by the seven microwave ovens and one convection oven—a testimony to the product that she endorses. There was no traditional oven in the place.

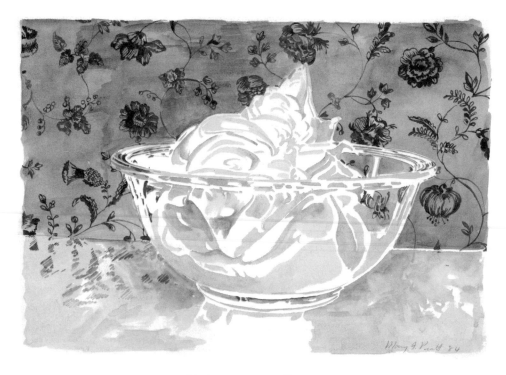

Meringue against wallpaper

Food in Quebec consisted of more than bearded men and skirted ladies eating salt pork and maple syrup in the bush. There was also a city life where people ate more lightly, usually only three meals a day. Breakfast might have been toast dipped in hot chocolate; lunch and dinner would include bread, soup, game, salad and fruit. Much was imported.

Today, the sophisticated food of Quebec's restaurants is considered by many to be the best of what Canada has to offer. Quebec attracts many young European chefs looking for their place in history in the New World. They come to Quebec because they know that their profession will be respected and they will learn and be challenged. Most are hired by the large hotels, and they bring with them techniques and recipes that are European in origin and formal in presentation.

Some of the older European chefs still prepare food in the traditional continental style. You can still find on menus dishes like Veal Prince Orloff, where at every stage of assembly the meat and stuffings are manipulated and sauced. Dishes like these formed the basis of classical cuisine, which some traditional chefs cling to with tenacity. It would be too hard for them to break out of the mould and combine sea urchin with asparagus, red wine sauce with a fish.

Though there have been some excesses as the younger chefs attempted to break away from restrictive rules, there have also been some brilliant discoveries. Jacques Robert, owner-chef of Au Tournant de la Rivière in Carignan, about a half-hour's drive outside Montreal, spends Monday, the one day he has off from the restaurant, combining various meats and sauces with an array of herbs to create the new tastes that lead critics to call his the best restaurant in Canada. Sometimes his efforts yield master-pieces, as in his stunning sweetbread pâté made with fresh butter and puréed sweetbreads seasoned only with a shake of salt and some grindings of fresh pepper. His onion confit, served with pâté or braised leeks, is made by simmering onions slowly with red wine and a shot of grenadine syrup.

Jacques Robert is a perfectionist and a master. I once spent two weeks working in his restaurant as a kitchen aid whose job it was to cut carrots and peel the quail eggs that were to be sautéed and folded into his spectacular dishes. He inspected my work piece by piece. If a carrot or potato's shape wasn't right, then out it went. And lots went out. I became so embarrassed at my frequent mistakes that I often ate them before Robert made his inspection. In one evening I ate two pieces of chocolate-hazelnut torte that crumbled when I sliced them because I hadn't sharp-ened the knife first; and two kiwi fruit because I had cut them on the horizontal instead of on the vertical.

I supplemented my underground diet with surreptitious licks of the sauté pans. I particularly remember a mustard sauce that he had swirled in the pan, then laid over some pink slices of lamb, before he tossed the pan aside to be washed, leaving just enough of that ambrosial sauce for a taste for me and the sous-chef.

I learned things in those two wide-eyed weeks that I still use today: that whole cloves of garlic, deep-fried in lard until the garlic's sting turns to sweetness and the soft meat just pops out of its skin is the best way, next to aioli, to eat garlic; that a cantaloupe soup made simply by puréeing ripe cantaloupe and adding, strangely, a bit of diced onion and a few drops of sherry gives a whole new meaning to melon. I will remember forever a dessert dish made by lining an ovenproof plate with fresh raspberry purée, covered with fresh raspberries, all pointing the same way and laid in a circular fashion, then covered with the whisked mixture of egg whites, Marsala wine and sugar called zabaglione in Italy and sabayon in France, then broiled briefly in the oven before it was hurried to the tables. Not one of those dessert plates ever came back to the kitchen with anything on it.

Jacques Robert is one of a group of innovative young chefs who, in the last few years, has taken posh restaurant food in Quebec out of the hands of the classically trained European chefs and redirected it. I had the onion

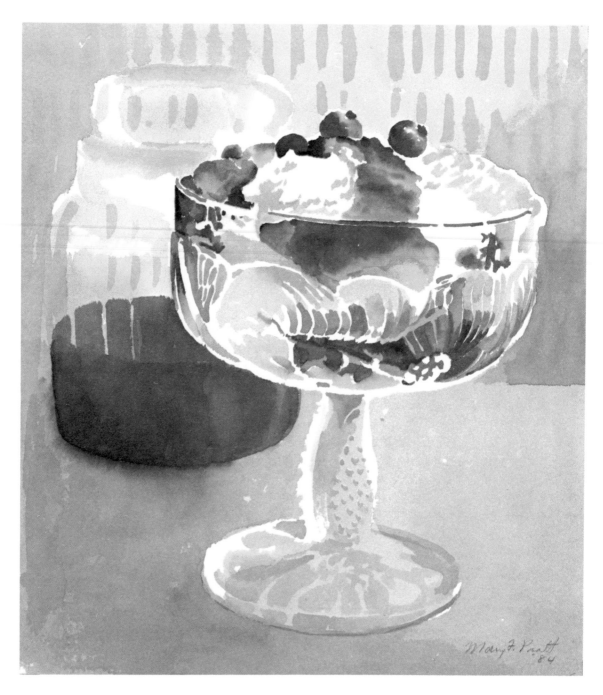

Blueberry dessert with raspberry sauce

This is our "patriotic dessert." The lemon snow
pudding, the raspberry sauce and the sprinkle of
blueberries make up the red, white, blue and yellow
in the Newfoundland flag. (M.P.)

confit for the first time in Carignan, though I now frequently see it on other menus. But the restaurants of these young chefs are where you'll first see dishes that are destined to become classics. Most of these new chefs are European-born, but not all are formally trained. What they have in common is new ideas and a commitment to serve food that fits with the times. If those dishes follow the rules, that's fine. If they don't, then the food overrules the rules. These chefs are all young, they all began their most serious work about five years after nouvelle cuisine became the rage, and they all insist on working fresh and working seasonal.

Though some of their principles are the same as those espoused during the rage, most of these chefs reject any labels put on their style of cooking, especially nouvelle cuisine. "There are only two kinds of cooking in the world," one once told me, waving his hand to banish overused labels, "good and bad." What counts is good food prepared simply, so that nature is the star. Vegetables must be served at a crunchy freshness, but not so crunchy that they're raw; fruits must be at their dripping ripest. The challenge for these chefs is in assembling flavours so that they blend, complement and provoke. Sometimes the combinations catch fire and you get something like the airy sweetbreads or lamb with mustard seed at Au Tournant de la Rivière. But sometimes they don't, and the results are downright silly, such as a withered bass steamed in an over-thick sauce of red wine and bouillon that I once encountered in a much-touted and shockingly expensive restaurant.

Keeping it simple isn't always easy. If nature is to be the star, then the best of nature must be auditioned. New fruits and vegetables are constantly being sought and, for the time of their fashion, placed on a culinary pedestal. Skinny little green string beans from Senegal have been popular in the last few years; so has lamb's quarters, a green that looks a lot like four-leaf clover.

To find such stars, the chefs must sometimes look elsewhere for the exotica that isn't easily found around them. Some turn to importing organizations which fly fresh produce in from Europe, a practice they feel they must embrace in their search for perfection. For example, in some fine Quebec restaurants you can sometimes find European scallops with their roe intact, a treat that elevates even the superb scallop. Fresh scallops can be had from the Gaspé region of Quebec, but when they are harvested, the roe is discarded. Eventually, if Canadians come to demand the roe, Canadian fishermen will stop tossing it away. For the best of local produce, the chefs scour the market, pinching eggplants, sniffing melons and examining the insides of endives. For many, careful marketing has replaced the sorcery of sauces.

Bee Macguire, the Montreal restaurant critic, refers to the core group of the young chefs who originally defined this movement as "Les Six." Besides Jacques Robert, they included Serge Bruyère of the restaurant A la table de Serge Bruyère in Quebec City, Alain Jourand of Le St. Trope in Ste. Adèle in the Laurentians, Pascal Gellé of La Chamade in Montreal, Guy Lafontaine of the former Le Mignolet in Mont Tremblant and Henri Wojcik, the Polish-born, inspired chef at Le Fado in old Montreal. These half dozen food philosophers form a kind of gastronomic think tank. They also have a very discerning clientele who expect a great deal from their restaurants.

It is the clientele that makes the difference in the quality of restaurants. Once when I was at Le St. Trope in the Laurentians, a regular client brought in a bottle of Château Haut-Brion 1934, cradling the wine in his arms as if it were a newborn baby, and challenged the chef to come up with a meal to match the wine. Though creative chefs work mostly for themselves, constantly trying to top their own last dish, it is the customers who allow and encourage them to do this. Such customers travel from restaurant to restaurant, simply to try the latest creations.

Sometimes creative chefs describe their menus to their customers in tantalizing ways. The recitation of the menu at Les Halles, one of Montreal's most popular restaurants, has become a ritual. It certainly adds to the drama and fantasy of indulgence when the chef takes the time to describe the trouble he is going to take with your dinner. At a restaurant in the Laurentians we were once handed wide menus and slim glasses of bubbling Burgundy to prepare us for the recitation. The chef joined us and described the menu item by item, dish by dish, listing the ingredients and techniques in such a compelling manner that I had barely settled on one, tasting it in my imagination, before the next one drew me to it. He told stories of savoury puff pastry surrounding the crunchiest of asparagus and the freshest of lobster; of a tomato soup that was simply a purée of fresh tomatoes with only a swirl of cream and a sprinkle of fresh basil to dilute it; of scallops offered with their roe intact, nestled in a sauce of fresh lemon grass and honey vinegar that had been aged in oak barrels. Though the chef recited the menu with almost a perfunctory air, to us the reading was poetry. We ordered lavishly.

Today some of Quebec's best restaurants are outside of the big cities. They are well supported, nevertheless, probably because committed diners in Quebec will travel anywhere to find a special meal.

The fancy foods made by dedicated professional chefs in Quebec can also be eaten at home, thanks to the abundance of the excellent food shops in Montreal and Quebec City. In the past five years these chic takeout shops have proliferated like basil after a summer's rain.

Browsing in the food shops of Quebec City is the best show in town, with all due respect to the Plains of Abraham. I have overfed myself on morsels from those shops more times than I care to admit. If the measure of the food in a shop is how long it survives the journey home, then the Mediterranean Epicerie scores high. I never get past the first stop light after I've left the shop before I've ravaged the brown paper wrapping and sampled the pizza niçoise or the couscous with its hottest of harissa sauces.

And there's more down-to-earth food around the corner, where you can buy Grandmother's cake (like pound cake with a syrupy topping), some terrific pâtés or sandwiches cut from four-foot-long French loaves filled with a selection of smoked meats. Along St. Jean, closer to the old city, is a store with wooden counters and sawdust floors that is laid out much as shops used to be a hundred years ago. Less formal but just as beautiful is the vegetable and fruit market in Ste. Foy where the freshest of everything is available. The best food shops in Quebec are like jewellery stores, with the merchandise no less revered and showcased. Fruits and vegetables are displayed as if they are to illustrate Boccaccio's *Tales of the Decameron*. Meats are butchered and displayed very carefully, each garnished on its own platter as if all that is needed is an infusion of heat to complete the dish.

Food societies are very popular in Quebec, and meetings and meals are well attended. I'm not referring here to the gourmet clubs formed throughout Canada by small groups of people who meet periodically in private homes to share camaraderie and dinner. In some of Canada's smaller cities, such groups have been formed to compensate for the dearth of good restaurants. But that's hardly the problem in Montreal or Quebec City. In those cities, there are so many restaurants that one just doesn't know where to start. The Chinese Dinner Club was formed in Montreal in 1976 to address this problem. Chinese food lovers, baffled as to where to find the best of it, gathered regularly at selected restaurants for banquets of eight to ten courses. The club grew, so that within a few years, members in Montreal and Quebec City were able to organize discounts at restaurants they try individually and on ingredients in Chinese grocery stores for the foods they make at home.

Quebec's food societies are formally organized large groups, with members who pay yearly administrative fees as well as top prices for lavish, formal dinners. Many have their own wine cellars, some with carefully collected stores that might be the envy of European monarchy. Some of these clubs, like the very established Montreal club, Prosper Montagne, are all male. Women, with their perfumes and distractions, are excluded, just as men with their noisy ways and cigars are excluded from the seven all-women clubs in Quebec.

The unofficial dean of all Quebec eaters is Gérard Delage, known affectionately as "M. Gastronome." "The food societies of Quebec are the most popular food societies in the world," he claims. "Even though people can eat very well in the restaurants here, they can eat even better in the clubs."

There are about thirty formally organized clubs in Quebec. One club meets every two months to hold dinners that break the rules, serving red wine with fish, or the salad before the meat. Others care more about the wine than the food. Most care a lot about both. Many of them hold dinners twice a year in large hotels in order to employ the services of highly trained hotel chefs who are only too pleased to have their attention diverted from their routine menus. The special menus are very special. Most are seven courses: a *dégustation*, or tasting of hors d'oeuvres and wines; soup; a fish course; a course of two meats: one fowl and another beef, lamb, pork or veal; salad; cheese, usually served with the evening's premier wine; then dessert, including petit fours and pastries; with coffee, champagne and *pousse café* to finish. These dinners are anxiously awaited and well attended, even at a price of at least $100 a head.

There are other unique foods to seek throughout Quebec. Sometimes they can be found in specialty shops, but sometimes they can only be found in their local regions. In the Laurentians, there is chocolate being made from goat's milk. Sea urchins, those darlings of culinary fashion for which one pays with the deed to the house in spiffy European restaurants, are being gathered in Rimouski. Farmers are experimenting with white asparagus and fiddleheads. In the Gaspé, if you're very lucky, you'll find cod liver pâté which, with its smoky-confit flavour, is as near to heaven as many of us are likely to get.

The legendary love of fat and starch that has produced delicacies like the pâté and the salt pork on maple bread, is also evident in Quebec's fast foods. There is no better place for junk food. Quebec, particularly Montreal, has some of the best hot and greasies in the land.

In Montreal there are the traditional *steamés*, found mostly in the pool halls along St. Lawrence Avenue. A *steamé* consists of a hot dog steamed in its bun, something like ball park hot dogs, so that the dog and blanket become as one. Just before the pool hall owner wipes his hands on his apron and hands the dog to you, he adds a large splat of cole slaw and some chopped onions.

I once did a tour of Montreal's best fast food places with author Seymour Blicker, who says that Montreal is the junk food capital of the world. He

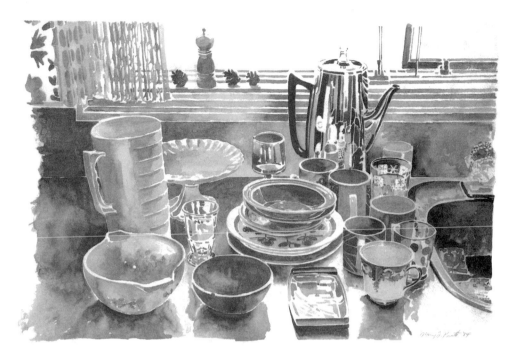

Dirty dishes

*Wonderful meals always end like this. But the
jumble of china, pyrex, plastic, stainless steel, a
wooden pepper mill and two pine cones is so much
like my life that it deserved consideration. (M.P.)*

took me to Patate Dorée on St. Lawrence for French fries and *steamés*,
claiming that theirs were better than the legendary ones at the Montreal
Pool Room, though I have tried both on repeated trips to Montreal and
would be hard pressed to choose the best. Whichever *steamé* one buys, it is
best to keep in mind this piece of insider's information offered by Blicker:
"You have to eat them right away when they're all full of puffy steam. If
you give them a chance to cool, they shrivel up and you can see all the
filler in the wiener."

Nearer to the area made famous by Mordecai Richler in *St. Urbain's
Horseman*, there are toppers, so called because just the top of the bun is
used as a carriage for hot smoked meat or salami. Montreal's bagels, made
in brick ovens, are compared to the best of New York bagels and are sold
even in Toronto, where people are chauvinistic about the local product. I
am very partial to Montreal's DeLalo burgers, made there with chilis long
before I could find them anywhere else in Canada. On my last trip, there
were morenos—stewy black beans and cheese on a tostada, found in a
Guatemalan restaurant in the east end. And there is always innovation: a

few years ago, Montrealers began to flock to pizzerias that prepare the pies in wood-fired ovens.

But you have to know where to go to find most of these foods. I once searched Montreal for days for the *poutine*, an amazing concoction of French fries, cheese and gravy which I first sampled in Vancouver, where some Quebec expatriates were selling it and *steamés* to curious Vancouverites. They filled a Styrofoam dish with freshly made French fries, sprinkled the fries with lumps of white Cheddar cheese curds, then poured a slightly spicy hot gravy over the curds. The gravy causes the curds to melt and so cements the three layers of potatoes, cheese and sauce into one. It is good and satisfying in the way only those kinds of things can be.

On subsequent visits, I have encountered the *poutine* many times outside of Montreal. At a country fair outside Quebec City a number of years ago, I discovered the *guedille*, a handheld version (and even possible forerunner) of the *poutine*. It was a hot dog bun filled with gravy-covered French fries. (Actually, the gravy was optional. Some of them, perhaps simply in a move toward some vegetable accompaniment, were covered only in ketchup.) The hot dog bun is different from the one with which most of us are familiar. It is flat-bottomed at the hinge, so that it can rest flat on the table, and it also holds more, almost like a boat.

Perhaps Quebec's best-known fast meal is St. Hubert's barbecued chicken, crisply roasted chicken with a side cup of very sweet and only slightly spicy barbecue sauce. It is run by Mme Helen Leger, one of the most successful female executives in Canada's food industry.

The interest in fast food has not escaped the hungry eyes of the Quebec government. In the late seventies it spent some time and money trying to develop an original Québecois fast food dish. Government-employed chef-chemists went to work and came up with a meat turnover, an apple turnover and a couple of other things. I tasted a few of them once, and they seemed fine to me, but apparently Quebeckers prefer poisons of their own choosing. The whole undertaking never took off and the project was shelved soon after.

It is unlikely that anyone eating in Quebec needs much encouragement from official sources. They might do us a greater service by providing austere retreats where we could recuperate from the excesses. You can eat your head off in Quebec.

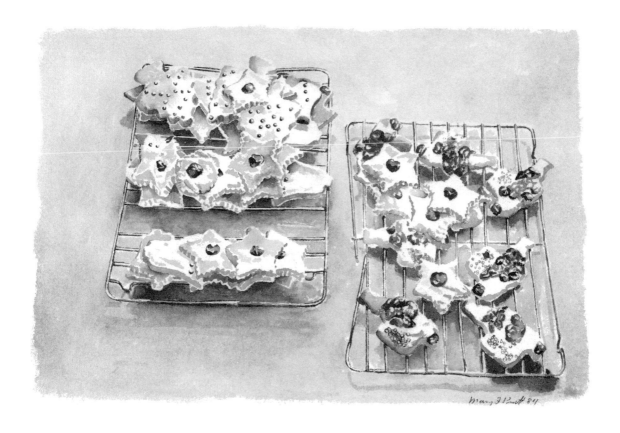

Christmas cookies

*These cookies were baked after a Christmas parade
and decorated lavishly by enthusiastic children.*
(M.P.)

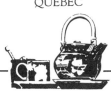

BAKED ENDIVE AND HAM

The Quebec endive is milder than its European cousins. Here each endive is wrapped in a slice of ham and the little parcels are baked together in a Béchamel sauce. Use a good-quality, lightly smoked ham.

3 Tbsp	unsalted butter	45 mL
12	endive	12
½ tsp	freshly ground pepper	2 mL
2 Tbsp	granulated sugar	25 mL
1 Tbsp	lemon juice	15 mL
¼ cup	chicken stock or water	50 mL
12	thin ham slices, with fat trimmed off	12
¼ cup	grated Cheddar cheese	50 mL
	Béchamel Sauce:	
¼ cup	unsalted butter	50 mL
¼ cup	flour	50 mL
2 cups	milk	500 mL
½ tsp	salt	2 mL
½ tsp	freshly ground pepper	2 mL

1. Melt 2 Tbsp/25 mL butter in a large covered ovenproof saucepan. Arrange the endive in the pan in 2 layers. Sprinkle each layer with pepper, sugar and lemon juice.

2. Dot the endive with the remaining butter. Add the chicken stock or water.

3. Cover and simmer slowly for 10 minutes. Let the endive cool.

4. Preheat oven to 375°F/190°C.

5. To make the Béchamel sauce, melt the butter in a heavy saucepan. Stir in the flour and cook over medium heat for 2 minutes, stirring constantly.

6. Gradually add the milk, continuing to stir as the sauce thickens. Bring to a boil and season with salt and pepper. Reduce heat and cook, stirring, for 2 to 3 minutes more. Remove from heat.

7. Wrap each endive in a thin slice of ham. Place in a buttered baking dish.

8. Cover the endive with sauce. Sprinkle with grated cheese. Bake for 30 minutes, or until the top is nicely browned.

Serves 4 to 6 as an appetizer

SUPREME OF DUCKLING WITH CALVABEC AND APPLES

Supreme means the breasts of the fowl, whether they are from chicken or, in this case, from the excellent Brome Lake ducks that are raised in Quebec. Duck is not a meaty bird, and most of the meat is found on the breasts. The breasts may often be bought without the rest of the bird.

Calvabec is Quebec's answer to Calvados, the French apple brandy. Fruit and meat are often combined in Quebec cookery, as they are in game cookery throughout Canada.

3 Tbsp	unsalted butter	45 mL
2	medium onions, diced	2
2	duck breasts, boned and halved	2
1 tsp	salt	5 mL
1/2 tsp	freshly ground pepper	2 mL
1/4 cup	Calvados or Calvabec	50 mL
1/4 tsp	allspice	1 mL
1	apple, peeled, cored and sliced in thick rings	1
1 cup	apple juice	250 mL
2 Tbsp	flour	25 mL

1. In a heavy skillet with a cover, melt 1 Tbsp/15 mL butter. Cook the onions until just transparent. Remove from pan and reserve.

2. Season the duck breasts with salt and pepper. Cook in the pan until lightly browned on both sides.

3. Add the Calvados to the pan and ignite with a long match. Let it burn for 20 seconds and then blow out.

4. Sprinkle the duck with the allspice, cooked onion and apple rings. Pour in the apple juice. Cover and cook over medium heat for 25 minutes.

5. In another pan, melt 2 Tbsp/25 mL butter and stir in the flour. Slowly stir in the gravy from the duck and cook for 3 minutes, or until thick.

6. Pour the gravy over duck and serve immediately.

Serves 2

—Perzow and Masson, Montreal, Quebec

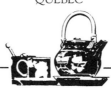

FRESH TURBOT THE BEAVER CLUB

Turbot is a large flatfish, delicate and delicious, which requires only the gentlest cooking and flavouring. This is a classy dish designed for a posh dining room where the powerful have their own tables and make deals on meals. The turbot is lightly poached in wine and butter, napped with a light sauce and served with julienned vegetables.

1	carrot, julienned	1
1	celery stalk, julienned	1
1	leek, white part only, julienned	1
1/4 cup	unsalted butter	50 mL
4	turbot fillets, approximately 6 oz/175 g each	4
1 Tbsp	unsalted butter	15 mL
1 Tbsp	finely chopped shallots	15 mL
1/2 tsp	salt	2 mL
1/2 tsp	freshly ground pepper	2 mL
1 cup	dry white wine	250 mL
	Beurre Blanc:	
3/4 cup	dry white wine	175 mL
1/2 tsp	tarragon	2 mL
1/4 cup	finely chopped shallots	50 mL
1 cup	whipping cream	250 mL
2 cups	unsalted butter, cut into small cubes	500 mL
1 1/2 tsp	lemon juice	7 mL
1/2 tsp	salt	2 mL
1/2 tsp	freshly ground pepper	2 mL

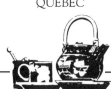

1. Preheat oven to 375°F/190°C.

2. Cook the carrot, celery and leek in ¼ cup/50 mL butter for 2 minutes.

3. Cut an opening in each turbot fillet. Stuff the fillets with the vegetable mixture and close the openings with toothpicks.

4. Spread 1 Tbsp/15 mL butter on the bottom of an ovenproof casserole large enough to hold the 4 fillets. Sprinkle the shallots, salt and pepper on top of the butter. Place the fillets on top.

5. Add the white wine and bring to a boil on top of the stove.

6. Cover the casserole with buttered parchment paper or tin foil. Bake in the oven for 10 minutes, or until the fish flakes easily with a fork. Remove the fillets to a serving tray or plate.

7. Meanwhile, prepare the beurre blanc by combining the white wine, tarragon and shallots in a saucepan. Add whipping cream and boil until reduced by half.

8. Reduce the heat and whisk in the butter cubes one by one until well blended.

9. Add the lemon juice and season with salt and pepper. Strain the sauce and gently heat until warm but not hot.

10. Coat the fillets with sauce and serve immediately.

Serves 4

—*The Beaver Club, Queen Elizabeth Hotel,
Montreal, Quebec*

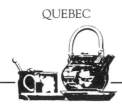

GASPÉ SEAFOOD CASSEROLE

This hearty casserole is a regional specialty in Gaspé, Quebec, designed to show off the excellent local seafood. It differs from seafood stews like bouillabaisse or cioppino because it has a sauce rather than tomato base, and because it has a cheese crust.

This recipe calls for different kinds of seafood found near Gaspé, but as long as you have a variety, substitute whichever fish and shellfish are locally available.

1 lb	fresh cod, cut in large chunks	500 g
1 lb	fresh salmon, cut in large chunks	500 g
1 lb	shrimp, peeled and deveined	500 g
8 oz	scallops	250 g
12	clams, shucked	12
1	green pepper, seeded and chopped	1
1	medium onion, chopped	1
2	stalks celery, chopped	2
1/3 cup	unsalted butter	75 mL
1	lobster, cooked, or 6 to 8 oz/175 to 250 g frozen or canned lobster meat	1
1/4 cup	unsalted butter	50 mL
1/4 cup	flour	50 mL
1 1/2 cups	milk	375 mL
1 tsp	salt	5 mL
1/2 tsp	freshly ground pepper	2 mL
1 cup	grated Emmenthal cheese	250 mL

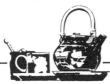

1. Preheat oven to 325°F/160°C.

2. In a soup pot, cover the cod and salmon with water. Bring just to a boil and then cook gently for 10 minutes.

3. Add the shrimp, scallops and clams and cook slowly for a few minutes more, or just until the shrimp turn slightly pink. Remove the fish and shellfish from the poaching liquid and reserve both the fish and the liquid.

4. Cook the green pepper, onion and celery in ⅓ cup/75 mL butter until the onion is translucent.

5. Add the lobster, cooking it in the butter for just a minute (the lobster can get rubbery if it is overcooked). Add the other seafood to the vegetables. Remove from heat.

6. Scald the milk by heating it *almost* to a boil.

7. Melt ¼ cup/50 mL butter in a saucepan and blend in the flour. Cook over very low heat for 5 minutes but do not brown. Slowly add the milk, stirring constantly with a wire whisk.

8. Add 1 cup/250 mL of the reserved poaching liquid and continue stirring over low heat until the sauce thickens. Season to taste with salt and pepper.

9. Combine the sauce with the fish and vegetables in a large, buttered ovenproof casserole. Cover and bake for 25 minutes.

10. Remove the casserole from the oven and top with grated cheese. Return to the oven and bake, uncovered, for 10 minutes, or until the cheese melts.

Serves 8

—*Michael and Marielle Sheehan, Gaspé, Quebec*

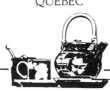

TOURTIÈRE

Tourtes were extinct tiny game birds that used to live near the Gulf of St. Lawrence, and were once the foundation of the filling for the original tourtière.

There are now at least two distinct versions of the pie. Tourtière from the Lac St. Jean region of Quebec is made with cubed meat and potatoes and is less well known than the dozens of versions made with ground pork or beef. Recipes for tourtière usually include savoury and ground cloves, which give the pie a spicy scent.

1½ lb	ground pork	750 g
1	onion, finely chopped	1
1 tsp	salt	5 mL
½ tsp	freshly ground pepper	2 mL
½ tsp	savoury	2 mL
½ tsp	ground cloves	2 mL
1	clove garlic, minced	1
1	bay leaf	1
¾ cup	boiling water or chicken stock	175 mL
1	medium potato, peeled, boiled and mashed	1
	Pastry:	
2 cups	all-purpose flour	500 mL
1 tsp	salt	5 mL
pinch	turmeric	pinch
½ tsp	baking powder	2 mL
½ cup	lard	125 mL
⅓ cup	ice water	75 mL
⅓ cup	unsalted butter	75 mL

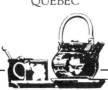

1. To make the pastry, stir together the flour, salt, turmeric and baking powder.

2. Cut the lard into the flour with a pastry cutter or 2 knives until the mixture resembles cornmeal.

3. Add the ice water gradually, blending it in with a fork until the dough is evenly moistened.

4. Gather the dough into a ball. Roll out the pastry on a lightly floured surface. Dot with the butter, roll up like a jellyroll to incorporate the butter and reroll to spread the butter through the dough. Roll the pastry up like a jellyroll again and chill for 30 minutes before using.

5. To make filling, put the pork, onion, salt, pepper, savoury, cloves, garlic and bay leaf in a saucepan and mix well.

6. Add the boiling water. Simmer, uncovered, for 20 minutes, stirring occasionally.

7. Remove from heat, stir in the mashed potato and cool.

8. Remove the bay leaf and skim off the fat that has floated to the surface.

9. Preheat the oven to 400°F/200°C.

10. Roll out half the dough and line a 9-in/1-L pie plate.

11. Place the filling in the pie plate and moisten the edge of the pastry.

12. Roll out the remaining dough and cover the pie. Crimp the edges and make an incision in the pastry to allow steam to escape.

13. Bake for 30 minutes, or until the crust is golden. Serve hot. (This tourtière tastes even better reheated the following day. To reheat, bake at 325°F/160°C for 1 hour.)

Serves 4 to 6

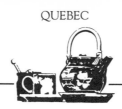

VEAL SCALLOPS WITH FRESH ORANGE SAUCE

In this recipe, tender veal is cooked in butter and napped with a sauce of vermouth, rum and fresh orange juice. The challenge of this straightforward recipe is in the preparation of the decorative and flavourful julienne of orange peel. The recipe includes no salt or pepper. If you are using unsalted butter and you prefer to include some salt, taste the sauce before you whisk in the cold butter and add a bit of salt and freshly ground pepper at that point.

4	oranges	4
2 Tbsp	granulated sugar	25 mL
4	veal scallops	4
2 Tbsp	butter	25 mL
2 Tbsp	dark rum	25 mL
1 cup	dry vermouth	250 mL
1 tsp	green peppercorns	5 mL
2 Tbsp	butter, cold	25 mL

1. To prepare the orange julienne, use a vegetable peeler to remove the coloured part of the peel (zest), excluding the bitter white pith. Cut the zest into very thin strips. Squeeze the juice from the peeled fruit and set aside.

2. Place the zest in a medium saucepan, cover with cold water and bring just to a boil. Immediately remove from the heat and drain the water. Repeat this procedure twice.

3. Finally, barely cover the julienne with fresh water. Add the sugar. Cook slowly over low heat for about 20 minutes, or until the water has almost evaporated. Drain and set aside.

4. Cook the veal scallops in 2 Tbsp/ 25 mL butter for 2 to 3 minutes on each side. Take care not to overcook the veal, as it will become tough. As each scallop is cooked, place it on a warm platter. When all are cooked, drain the pan of excess butter.

5. Add the rum and vermouth to the cooking pan. Scrape up any bits of meat that have stuck to the bottom of the pan and include them in the sauce.

6. Ignite the sauce and let the flame die out.

7. Add the orange juice. Reduce the sauce by half by boiling rapidly.

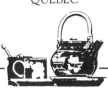

8. Add the peppercorns and the julienned orange peel. (If you wish, a pinch of salt and/or freshly ground black pepper may be included at this point.)

9. Quickly whip in the cold butter with a wire whisk. Pour the sauce over the scallops and serve immediately.

Serves 4

—Jacques Robert, Au Tournant de la Rivière, Carignan, Quebec

ONION CONFIT

If you love the smell of onions cooking long and slow until they are sweet and almost burnt, then this recipe should be in your collection. The onions are first fried in butter, then simmered in red wine and a bit of grenadine. The result looks like nothing but tastes like heaven.

This unusual condiment is based on a recipe from Au Tournant de la Rivière, one of Canada's best restaurants. Serve it with braised leeks, pâté or roast meats.

2 Tbsp	butter	25 mL
6	**medium yellow onions, thinly sliced**	6
½ cup	dry red wine	125 mL
2 Tbsp	grenadine syrup	25 mL
2 Tbsp	red wine vinegar	25 mL
1 Tbsp	granulated sugar	15 mL

1. In a large frying pan, melt the butter and cook the onions very slowly, until they begin to brown. This should take about 30 minutes.

2. Press the browned onions to remove the excess butter and drain the pan of the surplus butter.

3. Add the remaining ingredients. Cook slowly, uncovered, over low heat for 1 to 1½ hours, until the onions are very dark or almost black. Stir occasionally to prevent the onions from sticking to the bottom of the pan.

4. Serve slightly warm or at room temperature.

Makes 1 cup/250 mL to serve 4 to 6 as a condiment

—Jacques Robert, Au Tournant de la Rivière, Carignan, Quebec

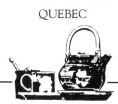

MAPLE MOUSSE WITH STRAWBERRY COULIS

The beauty of this maple mousse is that it's not too hard to make, not too sweet, and with its purée of fresh strawberries, it's very pretty. It was served at an international conference of food editors by a group of Quebec chefs at the Ritz Carlton Hotel in Montreal.

2 cups	strawberries, ripe	500 mL
2 Tbsp or to taste	granulated sugar	25 mL
1/4 cup	maple syrup	50 mL
2	egg yolks	2
1 tsp	unflavoured gelatine	5 mL
1 Tbsp	water	15 mL
1/2 cup	whipping cream	125 mL

1. Purée the strawberries in a blender or food processor, adding sugar to taste. Blend at high speed until the sauce becomes very smooth. Strain through a fine sieve. Refrigerate until serving time.

2. Heat the maple syrup with the egg yolks over very low heat, stirring constantly until it begins to thicken.

3. Moisten the gelatine with water, add to the maple mixture and stir until the gelatine has dissolved. Cool for about 5 minutes, or until the mixture has the consistency of raw egg whites.

4. Whip the cream stiffly and fold into maple mixture. Pour into individual moulds and chill immediately for at least 4 hours.

5. To serve, pour about 1/3 cup/75 mL strawberry sauce onto each dessert plate and unmould the mousse on top.

Serves 2 to 3

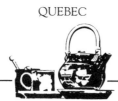

LEMON-GINGER SHERBET

In the midst of the long leisurely meals organized by Quebec's numerous food societies, a sherbet is served to refresh the palate. The sherbet, which is served in very tiny amounts, really just enough for a mouthfeel, is usually presented after the soup, fish and fowl courses and before the meat, salad and cheese.

2 cups	water	500 mL
1 cup plus 2 Tbsp	granulated sugar	275 mL
2 Tbsp	freshly grated fresh ginger	25 mL
1 cup	lemon juice	250 mL
4 tsp	grated lemon rind	20 mL
¼ cup	brandy	50 mL
3½ tsp	minced crystallized ginger	17 mL

1. In a saucepan, combine the water, sugar and fresh ginger. Bring the mixture to a boil, stirring constantly, then pour into a glass or enamel bowl (never use metal—it imparts a flavour). Let cool.

2. Add the lemon juice and rind. Place in the freezer for about 3 hours, stirring every hour until the mixture is semi-frozen or slushy.

3. Stir in the brandy and crystallized ginger.

4. Divide the sherbet among 6 dessert glasses. Freeze for at least 1 hour, or until almost solid (because it contains alcohol, it will not freeze hard).

Serves 6

PEAR CUSTARD WITH RASPBERRY SAUCE

The contrast of the sweetened raspberries and the creamy pear custard makes this dessert pretty to look at and wonderful to eat. Fruit custards sauced with a contrasting purée of fruit are popular in spiffy Quebec restaurants.

2 Tbsp	powdered gelatine	25 mL
¼ cup	water	50 mL
2 cups	whole milk	500 mL
6	egg yolks	6
1 cup	granulated sugar	250 mL
8	fresh pears, peeled, seeded and poached, or 2 19-oz/540-mL cans tinned pears	8
2 cups	whipping cream	500 mL
1 qt	fresh raspberries	1 L

1. Combine the gelatine and water and let sit to soften.

2. Scald the milk by heating it in a saucepan to just below the boiling point.

3. Combine the egg yolks and ½ cup/125 mL sugar in a large saucepan over low heat and stir briskly with a whisk until the mixture begins to form ribbons.

4. Slowly add about ⅓ cup/75 mL hot milk, stirring constantly. When the mixture is smooth, add the rest of the milk in a steady stream, stirring constantly.

5. Quickly whisk in the gelatine. Stir until the gelatine has dissolved. Remove from heat.

6. Purée the pears in a food processor or blender, or mash them and force them through a sieve. Add the pears to the custard and let cool for 30 minutes.

7. Whip the cream and fold into the custard.

8. Turn the custard into individual moulds or a large serving bowl. Chill for several hours or overnight.

9. To prepare the raspberry sauce, purée the raspberries in a food processor and strain to remove the seeds, or force the raspberries through a sieve with a wooden spoon.

10. Combine the raspberry purée with the remaining sugar. Place the sauce in a serving pitcher or bowl.

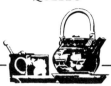

11. When the custard is firm, un-mould it by quickly immersing the moulds in hot water, then overturning them on individual plates, or spoon individual servings from a large bowl. Drizzle with raspberry sauce.

Serves 6 to 8

—Restaurant René Varaud, Montreal, Quebec

BLUEBERRY BEIGNETS FROM LAC ST. JEAN

This regional specialty of egg and flour dumplings boiled blue, sweet and unforgettable in a fresh blueberry sauce is much like the blueberry grunt of Nova Scotia. The blueberries of both regions are among the best in Canada and, if they are not to be eaten fresh off the bush, deserve this kind of cooking. The beignets should be served hot, with lots of freshly whipped cream.

4 cups	fresh blueberries	1 L
½ cup	granulated sugar	125 mL
2 cups	water	500 mL
2 cups	all-purpose flour	500 mL
2 tsp	baking powder	10 mL
½ tsp	salt	2 mL
2 Tbsp	granulated sugar	25 mL
2	eggs	2
½ cup	milk	125 mL

1. In a large saucepan, combine the blueberries, ½ cup/125 mL sugar and water. Heat slowly to dissolve the sugar. When the sugar has dissolved, boil rapidly for 5 minutes. Reduce the heat to a simmer.

2. Meanwhile, sift the flour, baking powder, salt and 2 Tbsp/25 mL sugar together.

3. Beat the eggs with the milk.

4. Make a well in the centre of the dry ingredients. Pour in the egg-milk mixture. Mix the dry and wet ingredients together thoroughly.

5. Drop the batter into the boiling sauce in large spoonfuls. Cover and cook for 10 minutes over medium heat. Do not peek. Serve hot with whipped cream.

Serves 4 to 6

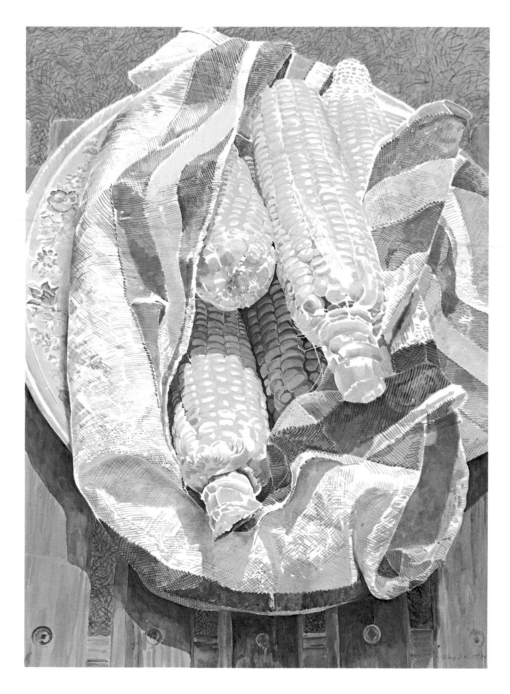

Corn in a Polish dishcloth

The lustrous corn, bursting with sweet fat kernels, so
golden, so familiar and so truly good in every sense is
a celebration of so many pleasant things. (M.P.)

ONTARIO

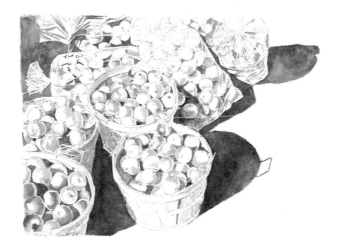

In northern Ontario you can get a hot beef sandwich, with enough gravy to drown your diet, or a plump roast goose and wild berry pie sweet enough to make your ears ring and your heart sing. In Sudbury you can get a plate of pasta and white veal; in Kenora you can get pan-fried pickerel and wild rice. In Kitchener you can't beat the pork and the peaches.

But in Toronto you can have anything you want. If you only have sixty cents to spend on dinner, on Tuesday nights you can have four chicken wings in hot sauce on the Danforth. If you have $500 to spend on dinner, you can do that, too, in a Yorkville restaurant that gives flamboyant gastronomes a choice between dinners of $100, $200 and $500 a person. With wine. You want strawberry vinegar, extra-virgin olive oil, no-name Dijon mustard or fresh white asparagus? That's easy. You want to duplicate the grilled sardines you tasted in Portugal, the pasta you put away in Pisa, the akee rice you noshed in Jamaica? A cinch. For those with a hunger for variety, Toronto means food in the fast lane. Within the areas that house Toronto's three million people, there are as many gastronomic regions as there are in the rest of Canada.

There was a time when Toronto had little to offer gastronomically. When I visited Toronto from Winnipeg in the fifties, I was disillusioned that one couldn't even find a decent perogy in what we in the West all thought was one of Canada's most cosmopolitan cities. By the time I moved for good in the late seventies, I thought I'd reached culinary heaven. In the austerity of January when I first asked the grocer up the street for a jar of dried dill to flavour a soup, he wondered why I wouldn't buy his fresh dill, lying in bushes on the counter beside the other fresh herbs. Next door to him I could buy fresh duck whenever I wanted and just down the street from there an array of fresh fish I could only have fantasized in landlocked Manitoba. And if I wasn't up to making the soup, roasting the duck or poaching the fish, there were dozens of places where it was ready made, and even more caterers who were anxious to make it for me.

The wonder of it all must have sent Toronto's natives spinning. For years they had tolerated, and even taken comfort in, its darkened steak houses and green-painted tearooms, like the Arcadian Court Dining Room in Simpson's downtown Toronto store, with its hushed ladies in hats and gloves, its pale green walls and slightly worn carpeting, its asparagus rolls and pot pies and turkey specials.

For years Ontario food gave the impression of practicality. It was a practicality so careful that it was often called prim. Suddenly, as fast as you could fry up a falafel, it was different. A wave of immigration in the sixties brought the spicy scents and rich textures of a dozen gastronomic communities, and the facts of fodder in Toronto were irreversibly changed. Someone summed up the change in the bewildered expression of an elderly woman, carefully dressed with a hat, veil and white gloves, who went into a downtown coffee shop and ordered her customary cup of tea. She was told that the restaurant no longer served tea, but espresso. With a bit of lemon, should she wish.

As might be expected, the change in Toronto's eating habits was prompted in part by the change in the liquor laws. In 1916, the manufacture or importation of alcoholic beverages was made illegal except for medicinal, scientific and sacramental purposes. Ontario stayed on the wagon for eleven years. Philosophical hangovers from the dry times made for odd quirks. A Toronto restaurateur remembers when he was not allowed to include wine in the meat sauces he served on Sundays. Years later you could have Burgundy on your beef, but it was possible to have a glass of wine whipped from your hands at 10:30 the same night. And there are still dry areas in Toronto, so that some restaurants, no matter how chic, must use quiche to define their sophistication.

When the change came, it didn't come easily. But change it did. Even Temperance Street in Toronto, which is rumoured to have been built on property donated on the condition that no liquor pass the lips of anyone on the street, now has several restaurants where diners imbibe freely, even after dark.

And though the changes might have been baffling in the beginning, they were soon welcomed with alacrity. The woman in the Toronto coffee shop might have balked at first, but before long she was inviting her friends to join her. And not long after that, they were trying to one-up each other with their latest finds.

These days the parade of people dashing from bar to beanery is the best show in town. Chic women so slender that they look as if a vampire has drained their blood, and hollow-cheeked men with carefully sloppy clothes make watching who's on the seats more fun than eating what's on the plates. In fact, these days in Toronto it's not really chic to eat at all. The city's slender beauties cannot take in more than Perrier and oxygen, burying the pommes Anna beneath the petit pois or slipping the sushi to the Samoyed under the table.

Now in Ontario's most with-it cities, the fashions in food are as fickle as fashions in dress. When hemlines last went up we were eating beef Wellington. When they went down, we were nibbling quiche. The Sanssouci restaurant in Toronto's Sutton Place Hotel runs ads in the newspapers offering their fall and spring collections—of food, not clothes.

Some of these culinary fashions are not of our own making. Toronto follows New York in its trends, and much gastronomic intelligence is gleaned through American publications such as *Vogue*, *Harper's Bazaar* and the W section of *Women's Wear Daily*. A few years ago when Toronto was still cuddling kiwi, New Yorkers were noshing sushi. The late Roy Andries De Groot told me then that the in-food was little salads made of squid—"You cut up the tentacles and put them on a bed of lettuce with a little vinaigrette." Within a year, Toronto had gone sushi mad and raw fish from bay scallops to sea bass tartare was on every stylish menu in the city.

Today, the taste for ice creams and funny-fruit sorbets has reached a zenith in Toronto. As soon as the last snowflake has vanished, the newest fashions in old-fashioned ice cream appear. Each year new ice-cream makers vie for the richest ways to incorporate chunks of chocolate and fresh fruit into frozen cream, giving established Baskin Robbins a run for its money. Indoors in both summer and winter, dessert parties are the thing. Lemon mousse, strawberry flan and hazelnut cheesecake are offered with Champagne—often by gloved butlers in morning suits.

In Toronto, where the food explosion in the pink-and-peach stylish emporiums has been nothing short of astonishing, the new waves of food seem to be created by very young people, some of them trained by the

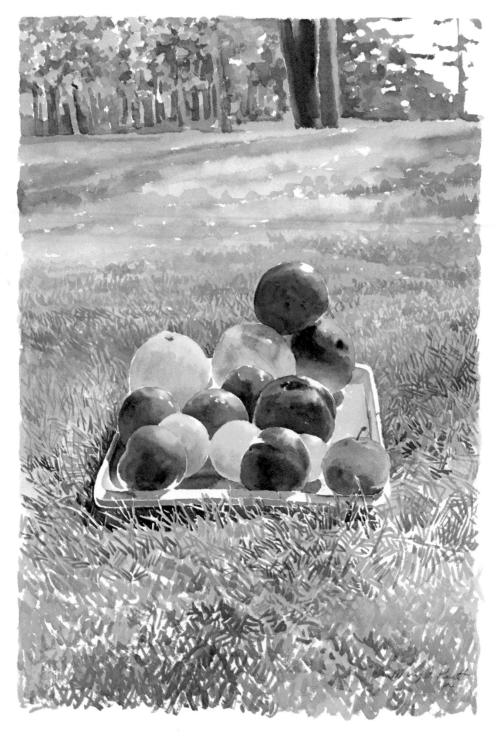

Fruit for a picnic

chefs' program at the forward-looking George Brown College. Werner Bassen was only twenty-two when he took over the kitchens at Fenton's and made hay with his emphasis on fresh ingredients manipulated in simple ways. Terry Seed took over the kitchen at the already excellent Hazelton Cafe when he was just twenty-six. Jamie Kennedy was only twenty-three when he began to combine scallops with ginger, making a revered name for himself through his efforts at Scaramouche. Mark McEwan, the chef responsible for the fall collections at the Sutton Place Hotel, was twenty-six when he began laying them in the aisles with his turbot glazed with butter sauce, his sweetbreads in strudel dough with wild mushrooms, and his chicken breast stuffed with scallop mousse served with carrot butter. Though most of his creations are accepted with alacrity, McEwan has had his problems with Ontario's "prudy eaters," who see his lamb in marrow fillets and fresh sage sauce and then ask if they can have a rack of lamb well done.

Though the rush to jazz up the dishes in Toronto has been welcome and in fact a lot of fun, in some ways it is a contradiction of the best that Ontario has to offer. There is a tendency to overmanipulate foodstuffs that are best left to shine with their own light. Toronto eateries have spent much time and money trying to be as good as the restaurants in Europe, while ignoring the bounty on their own doorstep. After all, Toronto gathers its foodstuffs from some of the richest agricultural land on the continent. Its eclecticism has been enhanced by Ontario's regional offerings: fresh perch from Port Dover, smelts from Georgian Bay, experimental produce from southern Ontario's government-supported Vineland, which developed square tomatoes a few years ago because they stacked more easily than round ones.

Ontario sends its prosciutto ham to New York, its Cheddar cheese to England, and its wild rice to France. Recently, the Rainy River Indian Band sent a twenty-pound bundle of rice wrapped in deer skin to the Prince and Princess of Wales for their wedding.

Ontario's current food fashions have nothing much to do with the province's ethnic mix. Food sociologists have been anxious to point out that the popularity of Italian restaurants has honest roots in Ontario's high Italian population. (Toronto has an Italian population the size of the city of Florence; Sudbury is a close second.) But most of the Italian immigrants are from southern Italy, where the cuisine is based on red tomato sauce and olive oil. Ontario's most spiffy and sought-after Italian restaurants serve the food of northern Italy, a more chic and affluent cuisine which, in fact, was the basis of French cooking. Ontario's luxury Italian restaurants are importing so many Italian chefs, that one is left to wonder who is feeding the folks back home.

The wave of Italian restaurants in Toronto has given restaurant goers a whole new set of worries. We had just begun to acclimatize ourselves to the bills of fare in fancy French restaurants. But once you understand the key words in a French menu, you have quite a clear idea of what you are about to eat. (There is an occasional exception, such as tripes à la mode de Caen, which requires some knowledge of geography, both of France and of the cow.) Italian menus are more metaphoric—and they are often chauvinistic. Many dishes are named for parts of the female anatomy, or make hungry reference to sex (those rascal Italians having long since noted a relation between the two appetites). According to legend, tortellini, the pasta that appears as predictably on Ontario's Italian restaurant menus as fettuccine Alfredo, were named by an imaginative chef contemplating Venus's navel. Pasta alla puttanesca is prepared "whore's style," purportedly because its quickie preparation using tomatoes, garlic and anchovies required little lost time between engagements, or because its heady aroma lured prospective clients. The menu language is flowery. A dish that is made with red chilis or cooked over a flame will be called "arrabbiata," which literally means "angry." A lovely dish of veal, cheese and ham is called "saltimbocca," which means "jump in the mouth."

The pasta craze, which has reached its zenith in Toronto and in Ottawa, has had some pretty silly incarnations in Upper Canada's restaurants. There has been pasta with prunes and pasta for dessert. But restaurateurs are delighted with it all. A plate of fresh pasta, no matter what it's combined with, sells for about eight dollars, at a food cost of about two dollars. However, though machine pasta may be better than the dried macaronis and egg noodles we ate with tuna fish and canned mushroom soup in the past, most is still thicker and more dense than it should be. I once had a plate of broad noodles made by an Italian woman on her kitchen table in Toronto. The pasta, which had been hand-rolled, was as light as air. I could see immediately how this angelic stuff could begin a meal without finishing the diner.

Sometimes Italian food is better outside of the city. Free from the demands of the kiss-kiss crowd, these restaurants are free to spend their energies on just making good stuff. The Italian food in Sudbury can be super. There is an Italian restaurant in Brampton that serves the best fettuccine I've ever had, by simply tossing a light spinach noodle with fresh cream, lots of grated Parmesan and black pepper.

There is also no comparing the spiffy Italian food of the brass and chrome restaurants to the food cooked in the homes of the Italian immigrants to this province. And the best place to sample it is at an Italian wedding.

I had known Italian weddings only by their reputation for the emphasis on food and festivity—a reputation challenged most notably by Jewish Bar Mitzvahs and Polish nuptials. As a result of the day and night I spent eating at an Italian wedding in Toronto, I can report with confidence that they are in the running.

The onslaught of food began only minutes after the kiss that sealed the ceremony. The offering seemed innocent enough: tiny tartini—little pizza-like pastries baked with tomato sauce that were served with drinks during the reception. The real test of stamina was with dinner, served an hour later. The first course was fresh cantaloupe blanketed with wide slices of freshly cut prosciutto. The plates were garnished with fresh imported figs, apparently a mandatory part of any festive Italian meal. Huge chunks of fresh Italian-style bread were passed around the table with each course; red and white wines flowed freely.

After some dancing and table-hopping, the second course was served. Green and white fettuccine, freshly made on the premises that morning, was tossed with a long-simmered tomato sauce and served by the bowlful to each of the celebrating guests. By the end of the wonderful pasta and three glasses of the red wine, I was almost ready to call a halt.

Next came the main entree. Each guest was served a platter that contained three large pieces of veal piccata, lightly dusted with seasoned flour, then seared and squirted with enough fresh lemon juice to empha-size the sweetness of the meat. With the veal came broccoli bathed in a cream sauce that had been flavoured with nutmeg, steamed carrots and a whole tomato stuffed with basil-dusted breadcrumbs. We were then allowed only a short respite before the next course. Huge platters contain-ing roast lamb, cooked sausages, roast rabbit and pieces of duck were passed around the table and each guest was coaxed to take lavish helpings. The reward for this abandoned gluttony was the salad course, followed by the dessert of tiny, fruit-shaped ice creams.

It was all a mere prelude to the sweet table offered a few hours later. The tables were laid in a wide arc in front of a five-tiered fountain and were trimmed with lace and decorated with large and lavish ice sculptures of swans and love birds. In between were gargantuan bowls of fresh fruit nestled in crisp lettuce leaves and a variety of pastries: cakes soaked with rum and topped with a rainbow of icings; huge bowls of whipped cream, homemade pies brought by friends of the family, and platters of cannoli, a traditional Sicilian pastry made of a crunchy case filled with sweetened ricotta cheese flavoured with rum.

But it just shows how limited your scope can be if you don't know what weddings to get invited to. Portuguese weddings, like Italian weddings, provide an array of appetizers and beverages during the reception. They also share the multi-coursed dinner. At Elizabeth Brianco's wedding in Toronto 280 guests began with a plate of lobster, shrimp and crab, boiled and served with mayonnaise. Next was "green soup" made from a purée of potatoes and broccoli. Then salad was provided for refreshment before the First Plate, or pargo, a wonderful Mediterranean fish baked with potatoes, seasoned with paprika, olive oil and served with rice. The Second Plate was veal, which was baked and sliced, flavoured with garlic, white wine, onion and bacon and served with mashed potatoes. ("We'd already had baked potatoes and rice, so I decided on mashed for the Second Plate," the bride explained.) Dessert was light—fruit salad or usually "just" pudding or ice cream.

Then, at about 11 p.m., came the course that separated the natives from the newcomers. No appetite trained on tea sandwiches and Perrier was a match for the gargantuan buffet. Guests were led to an enormous spread of shellfish and meats. At either end was a barbecued suckling pig. The inside meat was juicy and spicy with garlic and black pepper; the outside skin crunchy and very delicious. There were heaping platters of shrimp, lobsters and whole crabs boiled in the shell. There were barbecued chickens, round dumplings made from codfish and others made from shrimp.

And, not to be outdone by the Italians, this Portuguese wedding included a great number of sweets, including little pastries with custards, coconut cakes, beer cakes and bean and almond cakes. There were rice puddings and that particularly Portuguese dessert called Flan—sometimes also called "365" after the number of days it is served in Portuguese restaurants.

The marketplaces throughout Ontario are testimony to the variety of foods available in the province. The Portuguese shops in Kensington Market in Toronto have varieties of fish that one could only imagine ten years ago. Hot peppers, goat meat, odd fruits and odder spices, once totally foreign to the blandness of native Ontario cookery, abound in the Kensington shops run by West Indians.

East of there is the Greek area with its filo pastries and roast lamb and quail barbecuing in the windows. I also go to the area on the Danforth for

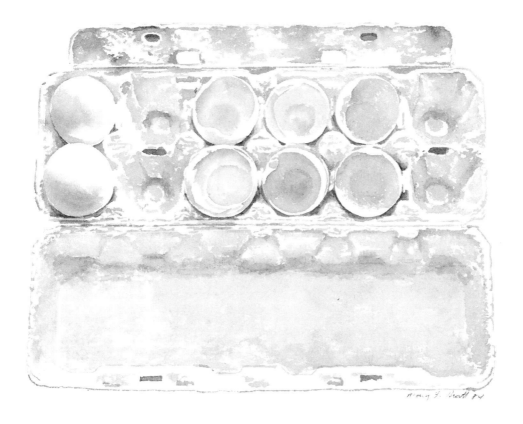

Eggs in an egg crate

*Sometimes when I prepare food, I'm so struck by the
visual pleasure it gives me that I'm not sure such
beautiful stuff is really meant to be eaten. Perhaps
we should, after all, concoct little pills to sustain us
and allow what has traditionally been food for the
body to become food for the soul. (M.P.)*

the sweets they make with almonds—especially those surrounded by dark,
bittersweet chocolate. And I have spent some very happy moments in the
restaurants that serve souvlaki, grilled pieces of lamb laid on a long bun
and slathered with tzadzicki, a powerful combination of dense Balkan
yoghurt and chunks of fresh garlic.

In Toronto's west end is the middle-European area with shop after shop
of sausages, strong cheeses and dark breads. In the city's huge Chinatown,
street after street has shops offering fresh lichees and Chinese vegetables.

Throughout Ontario, farmers' markets serve as more than outlets for
the fresh fruits and vegetables trucked into town by rural farmers. The

largest market in the province is the Ontario Food Terminal, which takes up miles of cement near Toronto's waterfront. This market begins the earliest of all of them, though it is open mostly to shop owners and some very keen restaurateurs. Markets like the St. Lawrence in Toronto or the Byward in Ottawa are city markets where one can get fresh fish and meat as well as the best of local produce.

The best produce is rooted in the enviable agricultural soil of southern Ontario. The Niagara Peninsula annually produces acres of luscious fruits and vegetables, including the vast harvest of grapes that feeds Ontario's wine industry. Ontario's marketplaces are showcases for this largesse. Maple syrup is sold in every conceivable form, from maple syrup candies to maple butter. For a short time in the spring you can find fiddlehead ferns and sometimes chanterelles. And there's always wild rice from northwestern Ontario.

In the fall, you can find the best of Ontario's produce trapped in glass jars, preserved for winter's scarcity. There are translucent jars of wild strawberry jam, gooseberry preserves, baby corn and pickled wild leeks. Squash of every shape and colour spill out of one basket into another, and you can buy varieties of apples—transparents, melbas, duchesse, greenings and snow apples—that are rarely seen outside Ontario.

Some enterprising marketers turn the apples into butters or cider and sell them alongside buckwheat honey or the world's most compelling gooseberry jelly, which is usually bottled in old baby food jars. By six the first sleepy urbanites are shuffling in—dressed in ski jackets in the winter and shorts in the summer—to buy what's going to become that night's dinner party.

It is a measure of the new interest in food in Canada that otherwise reasonable people who would no more rise at 6:30 on a Saturday morning than fall off a cruise ship, now freely leave their warm beds to argue the merits of brown eggs over white. For many, early Saturday morning shopping at the market has become a ritual. City streets that once were deserted now rumble with station wagons packed with leafy produce, sticks of bread and the wonderful bacon that was just discovered at the third stall on the left.

These keen shoppers might be best advised to buy the bacon at the Kitchener market or the nearby Waterloo markets. There is no better place to buy any kind of pork, smoked or fresh. The best spareribs in Ontario, if not in the world (with the possible exception of the White-house ribs in Winnipeg) are those from the Charcoal Steak House on the highway as you go into Kitchener.

Much of the wonderful food in the Kitchener area is made by the Mennonites, who first settled in Ontario in the early 1800s. Their cooking has much in common with their southern kin, the Pennsylvania Dutch. The Mennonite-German population has given Kitchener-Waterloo some of the best eating in the province, especially if your tastes run to filling, salty-rich flavours. The area even looks good when you're driving up to it. The hills start rolling; there are cows chewing on grass. Off the main roads people are dressed in black, turning horses and buggies into huge acreages of farms with pristinely kept wooden farmhouses and barns. The roads twisting up to the houses have wide, soft shoulders for the buggies.

Depending on the season, you may see wooden, hand-lettered signs at the beginning of these roads, which offer relishes and jams, fruit pies and summer sausages for sale—huge, long, dark-red sausages wrapped in a canvassy cheesecloth, with enough spice in them to turn your ears crimson. I make a meal of the spicy sausage, some of the dark bread God invented to go with it, and a very sharp Cheddar. It's one of those meals that you put all your strength into, because it requires ripping and tearing and heavy chewing.

All of these Mennonite specialties are available in the area's two main marketplaces. Those in the know swear by the rural farmers' market outside Waterloo. But the largest market is right in Kitchener, housed in an unlikely place for its farmland produce—the Eaton building. The market takes up a couple of floors and spills out into the back lane. This is a very well-used marketplace, so it's best to get there early, especially in the fall, when the produce is at its most lush.

Some of the goods that the Mennonite farmers bring to market is just plain produce, though because of its freshness, it's anything but ordinary. But the treasures I seek are those that you can't have unless you make them yourself: thick real sour cream, thick real sweet cream, the crunchiest dills and pickled baby corns. The farmers bring in shoofly pies, a sticky, gooey dessert filled with molasses and crumbs, shnitz pies made from dried apples and crumbs and a dozen varieties of breads and cakes. From tiny booths there are blintzes stuffed with prunes and cottage cheese. There is also an outstanding array of fresh flowers, cloth flowers, quilts and other handicrafts. Some local shoppers still bring their own baskets and bags, a reminder of the days before sellers provided them.

The best-known promoter of Mennonite cookery is Edna Staebler, who was raised in the Kitchener region and returned there as an adult. I can report that Staebler lays a generous table. She set lunch for us one day on the veranda of her home overlooking Sunfish Lake near Waterloo. She

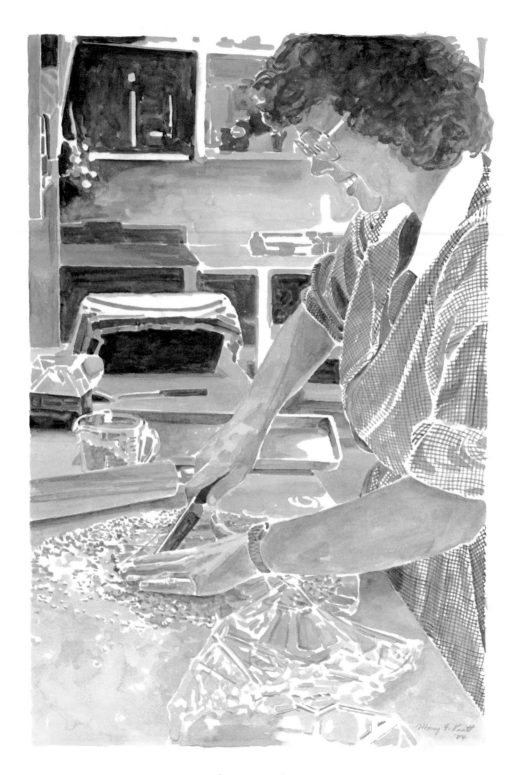

Cutting oatcakes

served a carrot soup so thick it could almost be eaten with a fork, and so sweet with carrots and salty smoked bacon that I had trouble not licking the bowl. She also served an asparagus soup that had a flavour earned only by the freshest of ingredients. Both were served with crunchy homemade crackers flavoured with onions. As the meal progressed there were more Mennonite specialties: hot potato salad rich with eggs; fresh spinach salad; a length of homemade sausage that had come from her favourite stall at the Waterloo market, some home-smoked ham that had been donated for the meal along with mustard beans, preserved beets and other relishes from Staebler's neighbours who had heard she was having a visitor from the city. Dessert was redundant, and delicious: huge bowlfuls of homemade caramel custard rich with carmelized brown sugar, whole milk and heavy cream. It was the kind of meal that people who work outdoors can still afford to eat.

The marketplaces of Ontario are a showcase for the best foods of each region, but travellers throughout the province have always found other favourite places to stop for specialties like Ontario Cheddar cheese. I think Ontario produces the best Cheddar in the world, an opinion supported by the New York shops that import and promote it. Near Ottawa there is Forfar cheese; not much farther, there's Balderson's, too. Such excellent cheeses are produced in small quantities by families intent on maintaining quality. A very few still make Cheddar from unpasteurized milk, so that the cheese is a living thing that ages and improves, like wine. Unpasteurized Cheddar is rare, but it can still be found at Leslie's Cheese House in Stratford or at Jensen's in Simcoe.

Aficionados try to buy Cheddar that has been made in June. It is richer because the spring grass on which the cows have been grazing is more lush (some feel that Cheddar, like wine, should be sold according to the time it is produced). Since cheese stores so well, it can be bought in large wheels or half wheels. Keep it in the refrigerator, coating the cut side with butter to seal it. Depending on how often you chop off a chunk, the cheese can last for months.

Another specialty of Ontario is its corn. Like Cheddar cheese it is best bought at its peak, though it must be eaten immediately. The closer corn is to the vine, the better it tastes, since the minute it is wrenched from its stalk its sugars begin to turn to starch. The purchase and preparation of autumn corn has become something of an eating rite in Ontario—a rite baffling to Europeans who have always thought of corn only as animal feed. In fact, it is only recently that Ontarians have begun to choose and cook it properly. Though the large corn with big yellow kernels may look the most appealing, smaller ears with light-coloured, small kernels are the sweetest. Make sure the corn is tightly wrapped and the silk is soft and moist. Loose wrappers and dry or mushy silk show an ear that is long from its mother. Pull back the top, check for kernels that are close together and plump. The kernels should squirt a little when pressed. And corn so carefully bought must not be overcooked: seven minutes after the pot has boiled is plenty. You can add a dash of sugar to the boiling water. When it's done, roll the ear in butter and sprinkle it with a touch of salt.

Collecting food is as popular a pastime as collecting antiques in Ontario. Along the routes that city people take to their summer cottages there are favourite spots for baked goods. Fudge brownies and homemade ice cream have been particularly popular, and there's hardly a small town that doesn't have a quaintly decorated outlet. Highways and side roads are dotted with ramshackle houses offering "old-fashioned" bran muffins, butter tarts and oatmeal cookies. Prompt an Ontario cottager and he'll tell you that the best place to buy scones anywhere outside of Devon is this little place just off the highway on the way to his cottage. Should these places be praised in print, they become no less popular than restaurants listed in the Guide Michelin. I'm told that the best pastry in the country is to be found in a railway station in Breckon, Ontario. The best southern-fried chicken in the province, according to a reliable source, is prepared by a cook from the southern United States in Point Pelee.

Ontario claims as its own the tart that has been called Canada's only indigenous dish—the butter tart. Versions of the treat may be researched along almost any route in the province. The tarts vary with the inclusion of currants or raisins, density of the crust and depth of the custard. Controversy on the etiology of this tart has been brisk in the halls of Canadian gastronomy, some of it provoked by those who claim it has Scottish origins. Toronto artist Charles Pachter has made a study of the Ontario butter tart his hobby. He claims that the best in the province—the slurpiest with the most tender crusts—are prepared at Wilke's Bakery in Orillia. This was no casual choice. For years Pachter held taste tests on butter tarts gathered throughout the province. He was so pleased with those from Orillia, that he had them bussed into his downtown Toronto restaurant daily.

I myself have spent as much effort travelling the province on the lookout for really good French fries. I have had my greatest success along Highway 7, which is strewn with fish and chip trailers. The chips become better until you reach Kinmount, where they are the best, especially when they're bought with the fish and doused in salt and malt vinegar. Home-made fries really are quite a treat in these days of oven-fried and prepackaged frozen ones. You can tell the packaged ones because they are all the same shape, size and colour. Not so homemade fries. Some are fat, some are thin and best of all, they're fried in real grease, which affects the chip according to size. Big fat chips will get only a crisp, light coating, leaving a soft interior. They have to be eaten fast and hot, otherwise they get flaccid from the steam. But little skinny chips will be fried right through, crisp and hard, and they always fall right down to the bottom of the bag, collecting salt and vinegar on their way. To my mind, they're the best of the bunch—worth digging down to the bottom of the bag for.

The food of rural Ontario is as hearty as the harvest—baked squash, fruit pies, cranberry relish—and city folks have come to appreciate it. This is evidenced by the popularity of country inns. Visitors dream of eating warm-smelling home-cooked meals in rose-wallpapered dining rooms; of four-postered beds where they can escape from the rumble of the city to the rolling green peace of the country. The emphasis on the food in many of these escape paradises is on the natural, the home-cooked, the comforting predictability of country heartiness. In the country inns, the apple pies are higher, roast beef and Yorkshire pudding are on Sunday menus and there is an emphasis on local produce. It's food that expects you have time to eat it and take long country walks to work it off.

One such dining room is operated by Gladys Fraser of The Spot on 7, a house-turned-restaurant on the highway just outside of Georgetown, about an hour's drive from Toronto. Fraser bought the home when she retired from her job as matron at a girls' school in Montreal. When you phone to make a reservation, you are asked if you want chicken, beef or seafood. The chicken turns out to be half a roast chicken, the beef, a gargantuan hunk of roast beef, and the seafood, an overflowing bowlful of lobster thermidor. But that's just the backdrop. The rest of the meal is a series of local specialties. First come the popovers, each large enough to cradle a newborn baby, put in the oven before your arrival so that they are ready for presentation a few minutes after you've sat down.

The staff are relentless. They then bring honey buns—delicious, coiled little yeasty buns sweetened with honey. With the meal come assorted relishes, varying with the season. The drink of the house is cranberry-ginger ale—there is no alcohol. Wholesome, filling food and clean drink.

Many of the country dining rooms are more citified and sophisticated, offering food more common to urban restaurants than to Sunday dinner at Auntie's. The menu at the spiffy Inn and Tennis Club in Parry Sound is the creation of Guy Urbin, a native of Dijon, France. Dinner might include shellfish mousse with lobster sauce and Champagne sabayon, or breast of duck in black currant sauce. The Arowhon Pines in Algonquin Park has long been known for its beautifully cooked Ontario specialties. And I once spent three happy days in the dining room of the Sherwood Inn near Port Carling, Ontario, because its exceptional dining room offers the best compromise between country wholesomeness and urban indulgence. You're inclined to dress for this dining room—in fact jackets are required for men—all the better to peruse the thorough wine list, and ponder the menu that may include veal with morels, cream of walnut soup and homemade preserves, muffins and breads.

Whether the food is taken from the city to the country or the country to the city, it's the blending of the two that has made Ontario tables—and eaters—groan with plenty. Trying to sort through the cornucopia that Ontario has become is no small task. Its regional flavour includes the tastes of all the provinces of Canada and most of the countries of the world.

It used to be easy to eat in Ontario when the toughest decision was whether the roast beef should be rare or well done. Now Ontario is a province where the answer to "What's for dinner?" could be "Anything you want."

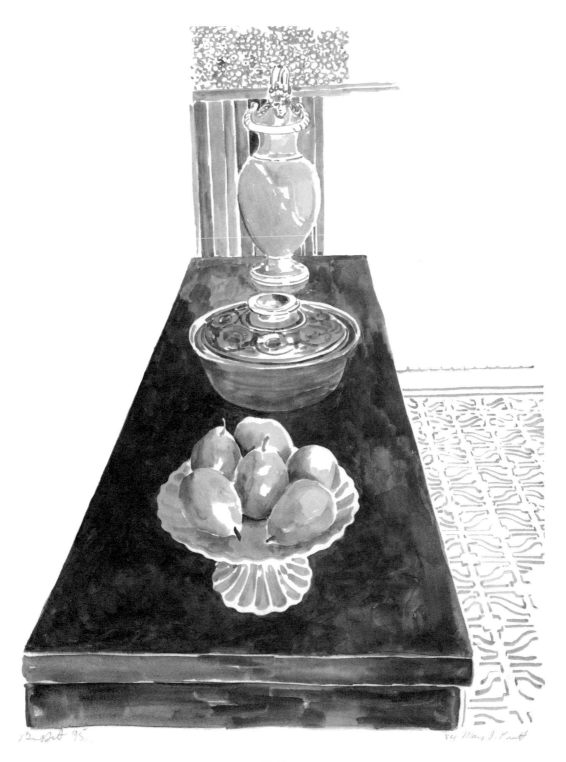

Buffet

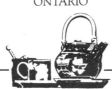

CHEDDAR CHEESE SOUP

Don't serve this as a first course. It is a meal in itself, and a delicious one, especially with fresh dark bread, a glass of ale and a green salad to follow. The soup is especially good when it is prepared with the excellent Ontario Cheddar cheese. Use an uncoloured, sharp, aged cheese for the most intense flavour.

4	slices lean bacon, chopped	4
1	medium onion, chopped	1
1	stalk celery, chopped	1
1	leek, white part only, chopped	1
½ cup	rolled oats	125 mL
½ tsp	freshly ground pepper	2 mL
5 cups	chicken stock	1.25 L
1 cup	grated Cheddar cheese	250 mL
¼ cup	cream	50 mL
2 Tbsp	chopped parsley	25 mL

1. Cook the bacon in a large saucepan for 3 minutes. Add the onion, celery and leek. Cook for a further 5 minutes.

2. Add the rolled oats, pepper and chicken stock. Simmer over medium heat for 40 minutes.

3. Purée the soup in a blender or food processor until smooth.

4. Return the soup to the saucepan over medium heat. Add the grated cheese a little at a time and stir until melted.

5. Stir in the cream. *Do not boil.* Sprinkle with chopped parsley.

Serves 6

CREAM OF WALNUT SOUP

The walnuts for this recipe should be very fresh, so buy them in the shell and in the fall, when they are harvested in Ontario.

2 Tbsp	unsalted butter	25 mL
3 cups	walnuts, chopped	750 mL
1 Tbsp	flour	15 mL
5 to 6 cups	chicken stock	1.25 to 1.5 L
½ tsp	salt	2 mL
½ tsp	freshly ground pepper	2 mL
1 cup	whipping cream	250 mL

1. Melt the butter in a 2-qt/2-L saucepan and slowly cook the walnuts for 10 minutes.

2. Add the flour. Stir to coat the nuts and cook for another minute.

3. Slowly add enough chicken stock to cover the nuts by about 1 in/2.5 cm. Simmer slowly for 1½ hours. Season with salt and pepper. Let cool slightly.

4. Add ¾ cup/175 mL whipping cream, then blend in a food processor or blender very briefly.

5. Reheat soup just before serving; do not boil. Whip the remaining cream. Serve the soup in bowls with a dollop of whipped cream.

Serves 4 to 6

—Sherwood Inn, Port Carling, Ontario

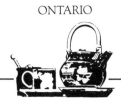

FISH SOUP WITH QUENELLES OF PIKE

This is a delicious clear soup, flavoured with white wine and herbs and garnished with light quenelles. Though quenelles (fish dumplings) may frighten even practised cooks, these are simple and foolproof.

Northern Pike Quenelles:

1 lb	northern pike, boned, sliced and chilled	500 g
1	large egg	1
1 tsp	fresh tarragon, or ½ tsp/2 mL dried tarragon	5 mL
½ tsp	lemon juice	2 mL
½ tsp	tabasco	2 mL
1 cup	whipping cream	250 mL
	Salt and white pepper to taste	
1 Tbsp	butter	15 mL

Fish Soup:

1 lb	fish trimmings, including head and bones of pike from quenelles	500 g
3	small onions, sliced	3
1	leek (the white and some of the green part), sliced	1
3	sprigs parsley	3
1	strip lemon peel, approximately 1 in/2.5 cm wide	1
2 cups	white wine or vermouth	500 mL
1	small bay leaf	1
8 cups	water	2 L
1 cup	clam juice	250 mL
½ tsp	salt	2 mL
10	peppercorns	10

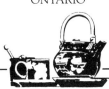

1. To make the quenelles, put the pike in the bowl of a food processor and blend, using on/off pulses, until smooth.

2. Add the egg, tarragon, lemon juice and tabasco and process until well blended.

3. With the machine running, slowly add the cream through the feed tube. Add the salt and pepper and blend in.

4. Butter a large skillet. Using two wet tablespoons, shape the mixture into dumplings and place in the skillet.

5. Pour enough hot water in the skillet to float the quenelles. Poach gently over low heat for 8 to 10 minutes, or until the quenelles are firm to the touch (the quenelles can be cooked in two or more batches). Remove the quenelles with a slotted spoon and drain on paper towels. Refrigerate until ready to serve.

6. To make the soup, place all the soup ingredients in a large pot with a lid. Bring to a boil. Skim off any scum that rises to the surface. Reduce the heat and simmer for 30 minutes.

7. Strain the soup through a fine mesh sieve, pressing some of the fish and vegetables through the sieve into the broth. Discard the contents of the sieve and return the soup to the pot.

8. Bring the soup to a boil. Divide the quenelles among eight heated soup bowls. Gently pour the fish soup over the quenelles.

Serves 8

—*Marilyn Linton, Food Editor,*
Homemaker's Magazine

COLD PASTA SALAD

It used to be that leftover macaroni was nothing more than that. Today it's a chic mainstay of Ontario summer menus. A good thing, too. Tossed with fresh herbs and vegetables, cold pasta can taste almost as good from its respectable place on the dining-room table as it once did out of a refrigerator at midnight.

1 lb	tortellini, fresh or frozen	500 g
4	ripe tomatoes, peeled, seeded and chopped	4
8 oz	Fontina cheese, diced or grated	250 g
8 oz	fresh spinach, chopped	250 g
1/2 tsp	salt	2 mL
	Freshly ground pepper to taste	
	Dressing:	
1 cup	vegetable oil	250 mL
1/2 cup	white vinegar	125 mL
2 Tbsp	Dijon mustard	25 mL
2 Tbsp	chopped parsley	25 mL
4 tsp	finely chopped garlic	20 mL

1. Cook the pasta in lots of rapidly boiling water until tender. Fresh pasta will take about 5 minutes to cook; frozen will take a few minutes longer. Do not overcook. Drain and rinse in cold water.

2. To prepare the salad dressing, combine all the dressing ingredients in a blender and mix at high speed for 1 minute, or until the dressing is the consistency of thin mayonnaise.

3. Combine the pasta, tomatoes, cheese and spinach in a large bowl. Toss with the dressing, add salt and freshly ground pepper to taste. Chill.

Serves 4 to 6

—*Bersani & Carlevale, Toronto, Ontario*

SPAGHETTI WITH SQUID

This is a spectacular dish from Joso's, an Adriatic fish restaurant in midtown Toronto. Squid and octopus are simmered in a rich tomato sauce, then tossed with spaghetti and garnished with fresh clams.

1 lb	octopus, cleaned and cut into 1-in/2.5-cm pieces	500 g
2	medium onions, chopped	2
2	cloves garlic, crushed	2
2 Tbsp	olive oil	25 mL
10	whole black peppercorns	10
1 Tbsp	Italian tomato paste	15 mL
2	bay leaves	2
1/2 tsp	thyme	2 mL
1/2 tsp	rosemary	2 mL
10	ripe tomatoes, peeled and chopped, or 2 14-oz/398-mL tins Italian plum tomatoes	10
1 lb	squid, cleaned and cut into 1-in/2.5-cm pieces	500 g
6	fresh clams, scrubbed	6
1 tsp	salt	5 mL
2 lb	spaghetti	1 kg

1. Boil the octopus in water for 30 to 45 minutes, or until tender.

2. Meanwhile, cook the onions and garlic in olive oil. Add the peppercorns, tomato paste, bay leaves, thyme and rosemary.

3. Add the tomatoes, making sure they are broken up. Stir and simmer until the ingredients are blended.

4. Stir in the cooked octopus and the squid. Bring to a boil. Reduce heat and simmer for 20 minutes.

5. Add the clams and simmer for a further 10 minutes. Discard any clams that have not opened. Add salt.

6. Boil the spaghetti to the *al dente* stage. Drain. Toss spaghetti with the sauce and serve.

Serves 6

—*Joso's, Toronto, Ontario*

LAMB SHANKS IN ANCHOVIES, GARLIC AND WINE

Well-known chefs often visit Toronto as guests of restaurants to prepare some of their specialties and teach their techniques. This recipe was prepared at Truffles restaurant in Toronto's Four Seasons Hotel during the visit of famed chef André Daguin of Auch, France. Don't be intimidated by the large number of garlic cloves. They become sweet and docile when braised.

2 Tbsp	olive oil	25 mL
6	lamb shanks, trimmed	6
1 Tbsp	tomato paste	15 mL
1 Tbsp	flour	15 mL
3	carrots, chopped	3
1	leek, white part only, chopped	1
4	onions, chopped	4
1	turnip, peeled and diced	1
12	cloves garlic, peeled	12
4 cups	dry red wine	1 L
12	anchovy fillets	12
3	tomatoes, peeled, halved and seeded	3
½ tsp	salt	2 mL
½ tsp	freshly ground pepper	2 mL

1. Preheat oven to 275°F/140°C.

2. Heat the olive oil in a heavy, oven-proof pan. Brown the lamb shanks in the oil.

3. Add the tomato paste and flour and continue cooking for a few minutes.

4. Add the carrots, leek, onions and turnip and cook for a few minutes more. Add the garlic.

5. Pour in the red wine and scrape the bottom of the pan to deglaze. Bring to a simmer.

6. Cover the pan and bake in the oven for 4 hours. Cool, then place the lamb shanks in an ovenproof serving dish, earthenware if possible.

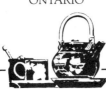

7. Garnish each shank with a cross of anchovies, 2 cooked garlic cloves and a tomato half.

8. Strain the sauce, removing the excess fat. Season with salt and pepper. Pour the sauce over the shanks and return to the oven for 30 minutes.

Serves 6

—André Daguin, Auch, France

SMOKED HAM WITH PORT AND RASPBERRIES

The hams found at the St. Lawrence Market in Toronto or at the marketplaces in Kitchener-Waterloo are superb. This is a variation on a standard baked ham. The port wine and raspberries combine to make a richly red and tasty sauce. The ham may be served hot or at room temperature.

1	5-lb/2.5-kg ham, cooked and smoked	1
⅓ cup	ruby port	75 mL
⅓ cup	brown sugar	75 mL
1 cup	fresh raspberries, washed and drained	250 mL
1 tsp	prepared mustard	5 mL

1. Preheat oven to 325°F/160°C.

2. Place the ham on a rack in a shallow roasting pan.

3. In a small saucepan mix together the port, brown sugar, raspberries and mustard. Heat slowly, stirring often until the raspberries are soft, about 10 minutes.

4. Put the sauce through a fine sieve to remove the seeds. Brush some sauce over the ham as a glaze.

5. Bake the ham, allowing 10 to 15 minutes per lb/500 g, brushing with glaze several times during the baking. Serve hot or at room temperature with the remaining warm sauce.

Serves 12 to 15

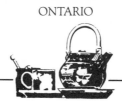

BUTTER TARTS

Some claim butter tarts to be the only true Canadian dish, although others imply that they have a Scottish heritage. Although these tarts are as rich and gooey as they should be, they're a little less sweet than most.

	Pastry:	
5 cups	all-purpose flour	1.25 L
¼ cup	brown sugar	50 mL
½ tsp	baking powder	2 mL
1 tsp	salt	5 mL
2 cups	lard, cold	500 mL
1	egg	1
2 Tbsp	vinegar	25 mL
	Filling:	
3 cups	brown sugar	750 mL
1 cup	unsalted butter, melted	250 mL
2 tsp	vanilla	10 mL
3	eggs	3
¾ cup	fresh breadcrumbs	175 mL
1 cup	cream	250 mL
1 cup	raisins	250 mL

1. Preheat oven to 400°F/200°C.

2. To prepare the pastry, combine the flour, brown sugar, baking powder and salt.

3. Add half the lard to the flour mixture. Using a pastry cutter or 2 knives, blend in until the pastry has the consistency of cornmeal. Add the remaining lard and blend until the pastry is the consistency of coarse breadcrumbs. Do not overwork the pastry.

4. Mix the egg with the vinegar in a 1-cup/250-mL measuring cup. Fill the cup with ice-cold water. Drizzle the mixture over the flour mixture and stir lightly until the dough is evenly moistened.

5. To prepare the filling, combine the brown sugar, butter, vanilla and eggs.

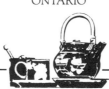

6. Soak the breadcrumbs in the cream and add to the sugar mixture.

7. Roll out the pastry and line the tart pans. Place a few raisins in each tart.

8. Fill each tart ¾ full with the filling. Bake for 20 minutes.

Makes 30 tarts

—Dew Drop Inn, Virgil, Ontario

DROPPED YORKSHIRE PUDDING WITH FRESH FRUIT

Usually served as an accompaniment to roast beef and seen at all the best Sunday dinners in Ontario, Yorkshire pudding becomes an inventive dessert in this recipe. It can be prepared with any variety of soft fresh fruits and served, if you wish, with clotted cream, yogurt or whipped cream.

1 cup	milk	250 mL
3	eggs	3
2 Tbsp	vegetable oil	25 mL
1 cup	all-purpose flour, sifted	250 mL
½ tsp	salt	2 mL
1 Tbsp	unsalted butter	15 mL
1 to 1½ cups	fresh strawberries and kiwi or other soft fruit	250 to 375 mL
	Icing sugar or maple syrup	

1. In a blender or food processor, combine the milk, eggs, oil, flour and salt. Blend or process for 1 minute. Let stand for 1 hour.

2. Preheat oven to 400°F/200°C.

3. Grease a 9-in/1-L pie plate with butter. Heat the pie plate in the oven until very hot. Remove from oven, pour in the batter, then arrange fruit on top.

4. Bake the pudding for 2 to 3 minutes. Lower heat to 350°F/180°C and bake for 30 to 40 minutes longer.

5. Serve warm, sprinkled with icing sugar or maple syrup.

Serves 4 to 6

—Ann Bartok, Toronto, Ontario

CARROT CAKE

This cake fits all of the requirements of a healthy dessert: it uses whole wheat flour, reduced sugar and no salt. Even so, it is the best carrot cake I've tasted—rich and full of flavour. The cream cheese icing is terrific.

1¼ cups	demerara sugar	300 mL
1½ cups	vegetable oil	375 mL
4	eggs	4
2 cups	whole wheat flour	500 mL
2 tsp	baking soda	10 mL
2 tsp	baking powder	10 mL
2½ tsp	cinnamon	12 mL
½ cup	chopped nuts	125 mL
1 cup	raisins	250 mL
3 cups	grated raw carrots	750 mL
	Icing:	
1 lb	cream cheese	500 g
½ cup	butter	125 mL
2 tsp	vanilla	10 mL
1 cup	icing sugar	250 mL

1. Preheat oven to 350°F/180°C.
2. Cream together the sugar and oil. Beat in the eggs one at a time.
3. In a separate bowl, carefully blend together the flour, baking soda, baking powder and cinnamon. Add the nuts and raisins.
4. Add the dry ingredients to the egg mixture, blending well. Mix in the grated carrots.
5. Grease 2 9-in/1.5-L round cake pans. Divide the batter between them. Bake for 30 to 40 minutes, or until a toothpick inserted in the centre comes out clean.
6. To make the icing, cream together the cream cheese, butter and vanilla. Add the icing sugar gradually until thoroughly blended.
7. The cakes must be completely cool before they are iced. Frost the layers no more than a few hours before serving.

Serves 10 to 12

—Naomi Berney Horodezky, Toronto, Ontario

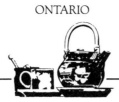

GRAPE PIE

The grapes must be seeded or seedless before they are wrapped in the dough for this unusual pie (dark Ontario Concord grapes are appropriate once they have been seeded). Serve this pie as a side dish with roast meat, with cheese for a vegetarian lunch or for dessert with lightly sweetened cream.

3 lb	dark, unpeeled grapes, washed and seeded	1.5 kg
1 cup	honey	250 mL
	Bread Dough:	
1 Tbsp	dry yeast	15 mL
1 cup	lukewarm water	250 mL
3 cups	all-purpose flour, unsifted	750 mL
pinch	salt	pinch

1. Prepare the bread dough by dissolving the yeast in the water. Mix 2 cups/500 mL flour with the salt. Add the yeast mixture.

2. Mix well and add more flour as needed, until the dough can be kneaded easily.

3. Knead the dough for about 5 minutes, or until it is smooth and fairly soft. Shape it into a ball and place in a greased bowl.

4. Cover the bowl with a tea towel and leave in a warm place for 1½ hours.

5. Punch the dough down and knead for another 5 minutes.

6. Roll out the dough to 1½-in/4-cm thickness and put into a 9-in × 13-in/3.8-L baking dish. Let the dough come up the sides of the pan and overflow the edges slightly.

7. Fill the dough with the grapes, pushing them into the dough slightly on the bottom and sides of the dish.

8. Set in a warm place and let the dough rise for about 1 hour.

9. Preheat oven to 400°F/200°C.

10. Drizzle the honey over the grapes. Bake for about 30 minutes, or until the crust has browned at the edges. Serve lukewarm.

Serves 6 to 8

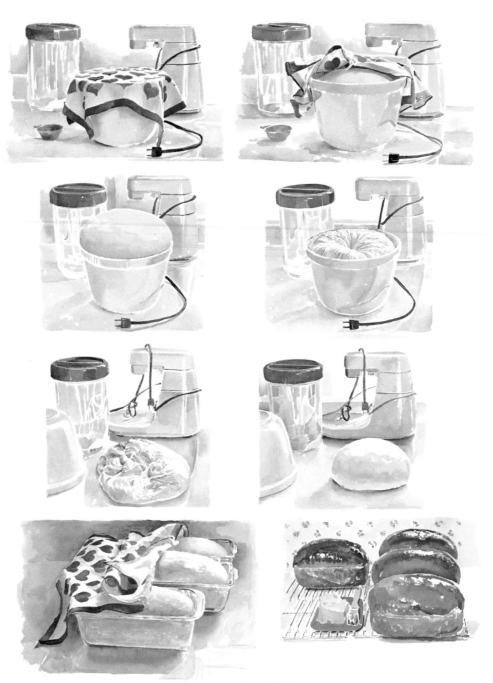

Eight images of bread baking

*I didn't learn to make bread until I came to the
isolation of Salmonier and had to learn. The process
has never become boring, every step is like a miracle
to me. It gives so much pleasure for so little effort!*
(M.P.)

THE PRAIRIES

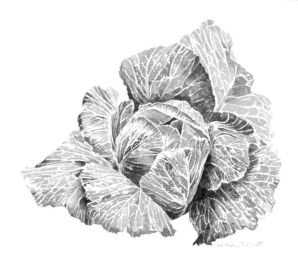

Let me put down my knife and fork and tell you how it all began. I started eating at an early age in Winnipeg and continued my gastronomic education throughout the Prairies until I was grownup and fortified enough to move my cutlery to Toronto. Since that day I have been forced to defend the excellence of Prairie food to my haughty eastern tablemates who seem to think of western eating as great amounts of heavy food that stay in the stomach for as long as it takes to elect a Liberal government in Alberta. "Great beef out there," they snicker, knowing full well that a plateful of red meat is low on the social order these days. Or, "What *is* a perogy, anyway?" they hoot, passing the sushi.

We who have lived Prairie food know better. Its superiority and variety is our secret.

Many people leave the Prairies when it is time to leave home, but they always take the food with them. In the Winnipeg airport you can often see boxes of City Bread waiting to be boarded on planes for Toronto and Vancouver. If you could look inside suitcases and lap bags, you'd find cookies and pieces of cake, cream cheese, hot dogs and, always, smoked fish, probably goldeye. My sister-in-law Carole always brings perogies—little pouches of dough filled with potato and/or cheese—because no matter how large the Ukrainian or Polish populations are in other Canadian cities, their perogies are somehow less delicate than those from Alycia's Restaurant in Winnipeg.

It is this informal culinary commerce that has spread Prairie flavours beyond the kitchens in which they originated. Throughout the years, travellers from Saskatoon have carried so many plastic shopping bags filled with food like huge cinnamon buns and butter tarts from Pinder's drug store, that an airline employee once dubbed that common carry-on luggage "Saskatoon Samsonite."

There are things to eat on the Prairies that can be had in other places, but they taste better on the Prairies. Chinese food couldn't be better anywhere than it is on the Prairies. Manitoba cream cheese is even better than Daiter's or Mandel's in Toronto. Smoked fish like goldeye and coonie are better on the Prairies than anywhere else in Canada, and smoked meats, especially smoked sausages and hot dogs, are the best in the world, Montreal included.

It's more fun to drink in Alberta than in any other part of the country. Alberta is second only to the Yukon in per capita alcohol consumption in Canada. Effete eastern drinkers may sneer at the mixed drinks of the West as they cradle their single malt Scotches, but they have never touched the inventiveness of the Alberta shooters like the Dirty Cowboy or Test Tube Baby, nor can they know the lilting joy of a gulp of beer and tomato juice, the popular Red-eye.

Perhaps one of the reasons that Prairie foods are such a secret to the rest of the country is that Prairie people don't promote them very well, even to each other. The best of the foods often stay cloistered within each of the ethnic communities.

The sausages are a good example of what I mean. The Big Boy sausage, for instance, is kept under wraps behind the counter at the European Meat and Sausage Company in Winnipeg's north end and is brought out only on request to those who crave its secret: clandestine chilies whose initial gentle tickle becomes an urgent roar. On the Prairies, sausage secrets are jealously guarded. I've always thought of it as part of a culinary conspiracy that hides from the general public (and certainly from any outsiders) the fact that some of the best foods on the Prairies are to be found in the sawdust-and-spice atmosphere of the tiny sausage houses and smoked food outlets that pepper the provinces.

The varieties of smoked meats and fishes are limited only by the number of groups producing them. If you want a Belgian-style ham, softly smoked with a nutty-sweet flavour, drive well outside of Winnipeg over flat fields to Swan Lake. In Ste. Adolphe, a largely French-speaking community in Manitoba, The Country Smokehouse smokes its bacon, ham and sausage country style, without nitrates. It also sells crackles—chewy-salty chunks of charred pork fat that feel spicily satisfying on the inside of your cheek.

The best-known sausage throughout the Prairies is the kolbasa. Eastern European in origin, it is a garlic sausage sold in rings as large as nooses and can be found in nearly every Prairie smokehouse deserving of the name. It is made in different styles (coarse, fine or buckwheat) and is often boiled and served with perogies. Eaten cold with dark bread and hot mustard, it is as fine a nosh as can be found anywhere.

You don't need much to accompany Prairie smoked fish, except maybe some lemon. Should the fish be pickled, it needs nothing but a chunk of dark bread to make it a meal. The best pickled herring I've ever had was made in Saskatoon and the second best was from the Oasis Delicatessen in Winnipeg. The owners wouldn't part with the recipe when I asked. Years later, a violinist, who prided herself on her ability to collect such tightly held secrets, slipped me what she swore was the recipe for the Oasis' pickled herring, and now I slip it to you. Wash 8 sugar-cured herring in cold water and cut into large pieces. Chop up 2 bunches of green onions. Mix up ½ cup/125 mL vinegar with ½ cup/125 mL oil and add 2 Tbsp/ 25 mL brown sugar. Alternate layers of the herring and onions in a large jar with a tight lid. Pour in the oil and vinegar and store the jar upside down in the refrigerator for one day. Turn it right side up and leave it for two more days. Then it will be ready to eat.

Many of these delicacies can only be found in their own communities. These are specific regional foods. Occasionally enterprising grocers will try to extend their markets, but usually the producers aren't equipped or inclined to supply for wide distribution, so these remain small, hidden treats. (One exception is the stunning smoked goose breast being produced in Manitoba and found in specialty stores in other parts of Canada.)

The tiny ethnic grocery stores are the best places to find the foods that reflect the ethnic groups on the Prairies. Like the Chinese restaurants that sold mostly pies and sandwiches, these stores have their treasures hidden behind packaged noodle dinners and cans of Spam. You can find almost anything if you look hard enough: Icelandic specialties, Italian, Filipino, Japanese. Because of the large German immigration to the Prairies, there are any number of terrific places in which to buy those sweet flaky pastries that turn afternoon coffee into a meal. The best time to poke through these stores is at the end of the week when the selection and hard sell are at their peak. Several years ago, one of these tiny stores even offered coupons toward the purchase of blue movies, with a minimum grocery order.

The culinary heritage of western Canada is so new that it can hardly be called a heritage. Manitoba, Saskatchewan and Alberta are barely

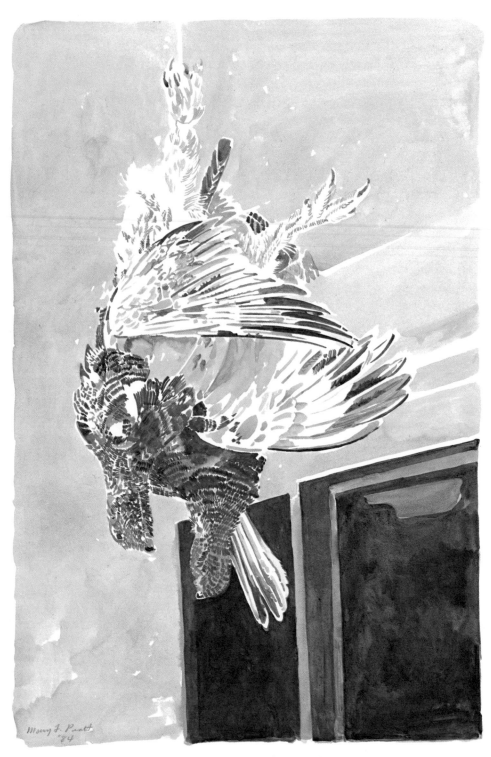

Partridge hanging on front porch

one hundred years old, and those years have been busy with immigration and population shifts. They have been pioneering years, and until recently the emphasis was on survival. The settlers who came to the Prairies were mostly of peasant stock. They worked hard in a harsh and unsympathetic climate. They didn't come to have dinner parties; meals were supposed to fill, fortify and break up the day. These are hardly attitudes that lead to a polished and sophisticated cuisine, or even a cohesive one.

Salmonella and other food poisonings were not uncommon during those early years, and settlers began to agitate for public health laws as early as the late 1800s. Although conditions improved enormously, the seeds of a germ phobia were sown and permeated the provinces for years. I can remember being taught to order nothing but a boiled egg in restaurants where I didn't know the kitchen, because "they can't put anything in it." Hamburgers were always under suspicion. You never knew what was in them and you could be cheated because there were too many breadcrumbs or poisoned because the meat hadn't been properly handled. When Salisbury House, the deservedly famous hamburger chain, began serving their sandwiches in the thirties, it was rumoured that they were called "nips" to avoid the suspicions surrounding the horrors of hamburger.

The effects of the germ phobia can be seen to this day. When exciting restaurants finally began to appear in Saskatoon a few years ago, a local columnist worried about germs. "It's great to see all the restaurants opening around town," he wrote. "What isn't so great is the concern of some members of the public about what's going on in some of them." He lamented waitresses who didn't wear hair nets and personnel who handled both cash and food without washing their hands in between. There should be more laws to protect the health-minded public, he pleaded.

When I sit at outdoor cafés in Alberta and Saskatchewan these days, I know how hard-won they are. There was a time when live plants were forbidden in restaurants because they might have bugs in them. It took years for people in Prairie cities to gain the privilege of sipping wine and eating lunch outside. When Winnipeg's first outdoor eatery was approved, health officials objected on the grounds that pigeon droppings might fall into the food. The restaurant finally got the nod from officials when it was decided that platters travelling into the filthy elements would be covered.

In those early days, nearly every Prairie city with a population of four thousand or more boasted a Chinese restaurant, a legacy of the Chinese who had immigrated to Canada to work on the railway. These restaurants were Chinese more by virtue of their ownership than their menus. Few had woks, and they got their supplies from companies geared to Canadian markets. These restaurants offered the kind of food they hoped the local

Caucasians would buy—everything from peanut butter and bacon sandwiches (at the National Chinese Restaurant in Moose Jaw, Saskatchewan) to blueberry pie. The pies were about as far from Chinese cookery as you could imagine. They were dense and gluey, usually filled with custard and canned blueberry.

At that time, few people ever considered ordering real Chinese food in Chinese restaurants. Claire Wodlinger, who as a child lived over a Chinese restaurant in Swift Current, Saskatchewan, reports that though her family often ate in the restaurant downstairs, they never ate Chinese food. While they were making their way through gravied meat loaf and bright-yellow lemon meringue pie, the Chinese family, cooking for itself, was digging its chopsticks into wondrous feasts that would not be accepted out front for several decades.

Now that we have taken the real stuff to our hearts, I regret that I live too far away to eat my quota of Prairie Chinese food. I wouldn't go to Winnipeg without a trip to the Mandarin Restaurant for their eight jewel duck: a completely deboned duck that has been cunningly reshaped, with a stuffing of chopped duck meat, pomegranates, spices and rice—the skin crisped in the roasting. And I wouldn't visit Calgary without eating a platterful of the Yum Yum Tree's ginger beef. Strips of marinated beef are heavily flavoured with fresh ginger and then fried in a sugary batter so that the outside crunches with sweetness and the inside is tender and perky with ginger.

Given descriptions of grotty roadside cafés and the pioneer austerity of the farmhouse kitchen, it might seem that the last place one would find white linen, polished silver and deferential service would be on the rough-and-tumble Prairies. Yet one had to look no farther than the splendid railway hotels in the midst of the dusty, struggling Prairies to find dining rooms so luxurious that any passing royalty might feel right at home in them.

The style and service were British, and the food, because many of the chefs were from Europe, was continental and quite formal. High tea was served in some hotel lounges (and still is in the Hotel Saskatchewan in Regina).

Meals in the dining room were served by gloved waiters and presented under those heavy silver domes one friend calls "tadahs" because that's what you feel like singing when the dome is lifted to reveal the platter beneath. These platters usually held roast beef with Yorkshire pudding or, sometimes, heated-up goldeye with a bit of fresh parsley—the gills garnished with a few lemon slices.

These splendid hotel dining rooms still exist on the Prairies and it is still true that they provide the poshest meals and service, where heavily starched napkins are routinely laid across your lap before dinner, and where the waiters are as starched as the napkins.

Freddy Nyquvest was for years the very proper headwaiter at The Factor's Table in Winnipeg's Hotel Fort Garry. The luxury dining room was done up like a wealthy Englishman's idea of a Canadian trading post, with a roaring fireplace, horseshoes, fur pelts and guns decorating the thick walls.

Like other hotel dining rooms of that posh ilk, The Factor's Table offered many dishes that were flamed at tableside. Freddy, who was an acknowledged expert with his much-requested Steak Diane, once actually set himself on fire and spent nearly a month in hospital recovering from the incident. In another hotel restaurant, the waiter set the entire table, and a few of the patrons, on fire. Everyone else in the dining room ate free that night. The enflamed patrons later sued and won. (It was incidents like these that inspired Winnipeg to pass legislation in the early seventies requiring fire extinguishers on the trolleys used for flambés.)

The hotels might have been wonderful at roast beef and Yorkshire pudding, but I always found the foreign-trained chefs crummy at handling the foods that were really indigenous to the area. (That, in fact, is another reason why the wonderfulness of Prairie food is such a secret—because the places where tourists eat the local specialties often don't know how to prepare it properly.) Goldeye, the West's sublime smoked fish, was grudgingly included on the menus at these emporiums, because a tourist might have heard of it and want to try it. But smoked goldeye needs no more presentation than to be offered at room temperature with fresh lemon. The hotels always heated it, presented it on beds of something odd and charged too much.

Fresh pickerel (the best of fresh fish anywhere, except maybe fresh cod from Newfoundland), if it could be found at all on menus, was ginched up with batter and put to sleep under a heavy sauce. Fresh pickerel should be treated with the care those dining rooms used to lavish on filet mignon— lightly sautéed in butter, garlic and parsley and served with a squirt of lemon.

It was the same with wild rice, which was always gilded to excess. If you want wild rice, here's how to make it. Rinse the rice well in a colander, then boil it in lots of salted water, as you would potatoes, for about 20 minutes. Change the water and boil for 10 minutes more, or until the rice is tender but not mushy. Toss with butter, freshly ground pepper and maybe some toasted almonds—if you must.

Both freestanding restaurants and hotel restaurants have changed enormously on the Prairies. Now they can compete in style and service with those in urban centres anywhere. Technology has made some of the difference—today you can have either Atlantic or British Columbia salmon in towns where only twenty years ago such choice would have been unheard of. There were three pasta restaurants in Regina the last time I was there, and now fish restaurants can be found all over the landlocked Prairies, where beef has always been the byword.

The light freshness of fashionable foods is a complete contrast to the Prairie inhabitants' fondness for offbeat drinks. And if the drink is ordinary, the name, whether it be the Barley Sandwich (a glass of beer) or the Red-eye (a glass of beer with tomato juice), isn't. Tomato juice-based drinks like the Red-eye, Bloody Mary and Bloody Caesar seem more common on the Prairies (particularly in Alberta) than in other parts of the country. The Alberta Restaurant and Food Association, in fact, claims that the Bloody Caesar was invented at the Calgary Inn. This, however, is apparently not Canadian enough for the operators of the bar in Terminal 2 at the Toronto airport, who substituted rye whisky for the vodka and renamed the drink the Canadian Caesar. Sipping this awful concoction, I hoped that no traveller on a stopover in Canada thought that this was the best we had to offer.

It's hard to imagine that such a perversion would be tolerated in Alberta. Bartenders in Calgary have told me that their patrons are very conscious of what goes into their drinks, and whether they're ordering wine or Scotch are very discriminating about the label. Patrons' creativity would be tested, though, with the very popular "shooters," the term used for the quickly downed jolts of aperitif—sometimes shot back two or three at a time—served in tiny glasses. Sometimes a shooter is made up of nothing more than Grand Marnier and not much different from the aperitifs downed in sophisticated cities all over the world. But usually shooters are much more interesting. There's the Dirty Cowboy made up of tequila, kahlua and cream; the Blue Monkey of crème de banana, parfait d'amour and vodka. Skid Row is anisette, grenadine and tequila. The B-52, made with kahlua, Grand Marnier and Irish creme, is by far the most popular shooter on the Prairies and has a flavour so well loved that patrons of Hopkins Dining Room in Moose Jaw, Saskatchewan, happily eat it in the restaurant's specialty—B-52 pie. Of course, there are dozens of other shooters, some of which, like the one called Orgasm, won't be described here. My particular favourite is the Ayatolla Cola, a murky mixture of tequila, rum, amaretto, kahlua and Jack Daniels. It's a drink that, like its namesake, shows no mercy.

In complete contrast to the hedonistic sophistication of the urban

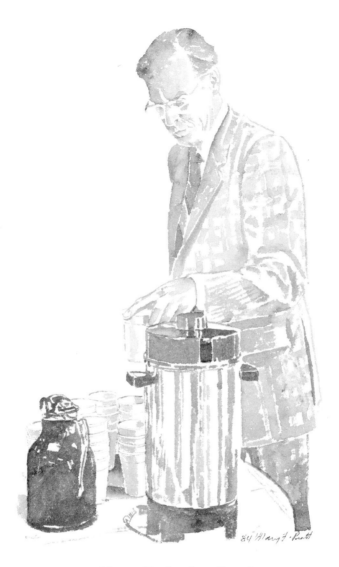

Vincent Tovell at the coffee maker

Prairie meals is the merciful plainness of some of the religious colonies, like the Hutterite colony near Camrose, Alberta, to which I once repaired to recover from a few Ayatollas too many.

These Prairie colonies are bastions of purity where tin cans, additives and anything that smacks of modern-day intrusiveness is refused. In Hutterite colonies the only food eaten is the food that is grown locally, and it is served simply and in abundance.

Much of it is produced for weekend farmers' markets, so the Friday afternoon I was in Camrose for lunch, I found most of the activity devoted to cleaning and bagging fresh vegetables for market. The colony is located deep in the countryside. Entirely self-sufficient, it has its own food supply, its own electricity and, most important, its own self-contained society. I walked through the scrubbed chapel, through homes, classrooms and through the shining, stainless-steel kitchens. There were countless store-rooms lined with preserves and a huge barn filled with bins of fresh vegetables being cleaned and sorted by young girls.

Members of the colony are called to the dining hall by a bell. The men file into one side of the austere room, the women into the other. The long Arborite tables are filled with plates of freshly made bread, pots of butter, dishes of new potatoes, cucumbers (both fresh and preserved), tomatoes and radish salad. My hostess motions to jars filled with cutlery and suggests that I "take some tools." There are a great many hot dishes: huge chunks of roast ham, platters of roast chicken and bowls piled high with steaming buckwheat. And this is just lunch.

When I protest at the second helping being heaped on my plate, I'm told, "If you're not still hungry, you haven't worked hard enough today." I eat more.

Basic foodstuffs like those served on the Hutterite colony are what is best known about the Prairies. Less well acknowledged is that Prairie baking is among the best in a country that's known for its baking.

Food made with flour should taste good here. The Prairies are the breadbasket of Canada, and the best bread is Winnipeg's City Bread. Though there are many theories on what makes it special, the consensus is that, during the baking process, steam is forced into the oven to give the bread crust extra crispness and the inside extra chewiness.

Why is baking on the Prairies so much better than elsewhere in this country? After all, everyone in Canada uses the same flour. Maybe it is better because it is taken so much more seriously there. On the Prairies, baking is the measure of real prowess.

No one ever calls it anything but "baking," though, in fact, many of the things aren't actually baked. There are wondrous mixtures of maraschino cherries, chocolate chips, miniature marshmallows and nuts. They are most cherished at teas, Bar Mitzvahs and funerals—the daintiest on display in three-tiered dishes called comports.

Most of these concoctions sound as if they have been named by three-year-olds. Hello Dollies are a mixture of chocolate chips, nuts and coconut; Yum Yums are made with Graham wafers, chocolate chips, walnuts and condensed milk; Pineapple Delights are egg whites, vanilla and canned pineapple cubes. My personal favourites were Melting Moments, which are nothing more than a bite of egg white meringue with an almond in the centre. They do, in fact, melt in your mouth in a moment, leaving time and appetite for Roly Poly, made with Turkish Delight, nuts, jam, coconut and icing sugar.

The Bar Mitzvah sweet tables on the Prairies have displays of every known pastry served up with a style and in amounts that I have seen nowhere else in Canada. The sweet table is not a phenomenon known only to Bar Mitzvah guests—other groups have long enjoyed the pleasure of a course, separated by a few hours from all the others, dedicated solely to eye appeal and the deliciousness of sweet things. You see the same things at Italian and Portuguese weddings in Toronto, and the current fashion for dessert parties is an attempt to capture the sweet table's grandeur. But nowhere have I witnessed the variety and sheer largesse of those in Prairie cities.

An average sweet table includes three different kinds of cheesecake (cherry topping, blueberry topping and one combined in some way with chocolate). Prairie cheesecake can bring you to your knees, if not to your own funeral, because it is made only with the rich local cream cheese, eggs, sugar, maybe sour cream and whatever topping or flavouring makes that particular recipe unique. No Prairie cheesecake ever contains gelatine.

There will be at least a few tortes, always including mocha or chocolate, made up of at least five layers, each of which takes an age to make (though custom dictates that the baker dismiss each creation as "a cinch" to prepare). The layers are bonded by fillings such as hazelnut, chocolate or custard, and the whole tower is coated with some variant of frosting. Tortes are always heavily decorated with diddles and doodads, and more than one baker has made her reputation solely on the originality of her icing.

While the sweet tables I remember from my adolescence featured tortes and dainties, today's dessert spreads are known by their chocolate. This dark confection has replaced chopped liver as a sculpting medium at parties. Chocolate is formed into leaves, branches and figures. A frequent sight is the chocolate "paper" bag, which is formed by smearing melted chocolate on the outside of an oiled lunch bag; the paper is later removed and the resultant chocolate container filled with fresh fruits or confections so that the effect is one of a chocolate cornucopia.

There are always platters of fresh fruit on a sweet table: strawberries, melons, fresh pineapple and grapes. They are largely for colour, or for guests on diets, including those who feel that the addition of a few pieces of fruit to a plate filled with various iced and custarded cakes gives some evidence that self-control is being exercised.

Baking recipes are best gleaned from the little community cookbooks produced in profusion throughout western Canada, where every baker

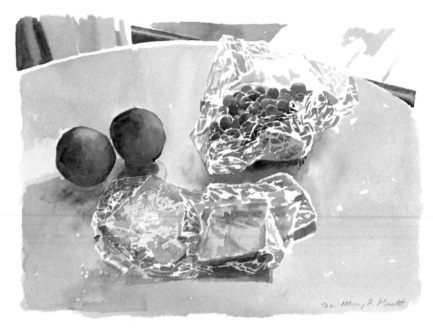

School lunch

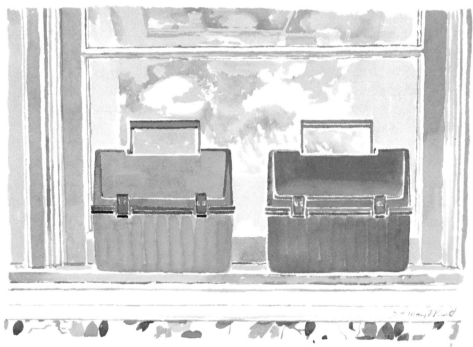

Lunch boxes

*I tried to be inventive about lunches,
but the children didn't want hot soup and carrot
sticks. They wanted orange juice and peanut butter
sandwiches. Always. (M.P.)*

has her own reputation. "All you need to do to know about whether a recipe is any good is to read the name on the bottom," one Winnipegger told me with assurance. "If that's Mrs. Smolinsky's cheesecake, it's good. But if it's Mrs. Robinson's, watch for gelatine."

Some are more than just cookery books. They offer hints that keep Prairie households going. In *The Centennial Cookbook* published in 1966, Anne Leatherdale of Saskatoon suggests that the reader try cooking beets in coffee and "you'll never want them any other way."

Cookbooks are a particular phenomenon of Alberta and Saskatchewan. There, aspiring authors have put out dozens of them, many self-published. It is estimated that it costs about $30,000 to publish a cookbook on one's own, and some women have pooled their life savings in order to do so.

These cookbook authors have been inspired by more than pioneer spirit. Everyone yearns for the success of *The Best of Bridge*. It was conceived in 1975 by a group of eight Calgary women looking for something besides bridge to fill their afternoons. They put together their favourite recipes while their husbands chuckled about "the cute little project." The husbands soon stopped chuckling as first-year sales of the book reached $1.1 million.

Sequels have kept the eight women chuckling and others inspired; anyone with a remote interest in cooking has jumped on the bandwagon and books by such esoteric groups as the Josephburg Alberta Men's Choir have been published. Riffling through the books, you'll find recipes for tuna casserole with pecans, creamed chicken with sherry, jellied salads and usually something called Night Before Casserole.

Gatherings, especially around food, have always helped to allay the long winters and relieve the isolated tedium of Prairie living. And the joy that Prairie folk cling to during those few short weeks between winters is a sort of midsummer madness. In Manitoba there are frog-jumping contests and other skill-testing challenges that would never take place in the depths of winter when outdoors is the last place you would want to be. People will try things in the summer that they would never think of at other times of the year. I travelled across a scorched Saskatchewan Prairie one July day to have my pizza read by a poet who claimed that pizza pies can be read in the same way that tea leaves are read, and that the way you eat a pizza reveals the secrets of your character.

During the summer, Edmonton has its Heritage Days, Calgary its Stampede and Manitoba its Icelandic Festival and Folklorama. The best part of these festivals is the celebration of ethnic food and drink. At Folklorama in Winnipeg, celebrants teeter from pavilion to pavilion, as intent on the food and drink as on the dancing and handicrafts.

In Saskatchewan one summer, I found myself a participant in the World Cabbage Roll Eating Contest, held annually by the O & O Drive In in Saskatoon. A cabbage roll is made by filling a steamed cabbage leaf with a mixture of ground meat and rice. The rolls, usually about the size and shape of huge Cuban cigars, are then braised in tomato sauce.

The contest was part of the Louis Riel Day festivities. It is worth describing because it is very popular and shows, I think, the remarkable stamina that helped make this country great. In the first heat, each contestant is presented with two pounds of cabbage rolls. They must be consumed in two minutes flat. The winners, if they can be considered such, go on to the final heat, the winner of which is declared world champion.

Cabbage rolls are not easy to eat at any time, and at top speed they're pretty daunting. The sauce acts as a lubricant to ensure safe passage down the gullet. But swallowing them isn't the only challenge; the stomach then has the responsibility of processing the concoction. Under ideal circumstances, the rolls are eaten with a knife and fork and chewed carefully because of the bulk of the rice and the fibre of the cabbage. But, as the only woman on a five-person panel, I had no such luxury. With a gun blast, the race was on.

It was immediately apparent that chewing was a waste of time. I tried to swallow the holubsi whole, but the first one stuck halfway down and I had to force subsequent rolls past the one immobilized in my throat. In what felt like three hours but was really only two minutes, the race was over. The winner, Tony Pistun of Foxford, Saskatchewan, went on to win the championship. Including the first heat, he consumed a total of four pounds of cabbage rolls in less than four minutes.

It looked as if Tony had spent a lifetime training for such events. He is well over six feet tall and weighs nearly three hundred pounds. I interviewed him the next morning at his sister's house in Saskatoon, where I was served the best pancakes I have ever had. They are a cinch. Mix 1 1/2 cups/375 mL flour (any kind—whole wheat, unbleached, all-purpose) with 1 Tbsp/15 mL baking powder, 1 tsp/5 mL salt, 4 beaten eggs and 1 1/4 cups/300 mL milk. Don't overmix or they'll become tough. It's okay if there are lumps in the batter. You can add some fresh blueberries or Saskatoonberries at this point, if you wish. Fry the pancakes on a hot griddle in just a smear of butter.

Many nations have ways of giftwrapping little bits of leftovers and making a new dish out of them. The Italians wrap up some chopped

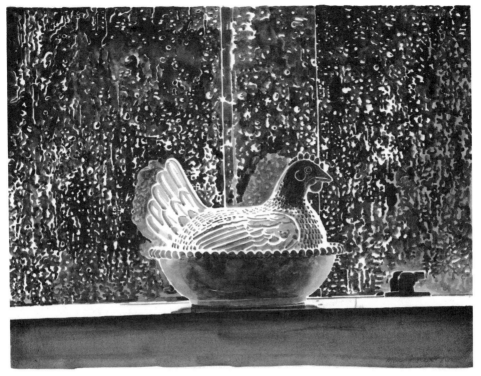

China hen—rainy window

*I particularly like this image of the white china hen
against a rainy night window, its shape is almost
mirrored by the window, its reflection pale against
the night's black. (M.P.)*

veal and call it ravioli; the Chinese have their wontons and the Indians
their samosas. Usually the leftover is meat, a valuable food in any country.
I've always thought it a particular comment on the penury and resource-
fulness of the folks who settled the Prairies that the treasure they have
chosen to extend is the leftover potato. It is wrapped up in dough and
called a perogy.

My eastern tablemates consider the perogy a metaphor for "fortifying"
Prairie cuisine. This is, I think, a short-sighted view. They have had
inadequate exposure to the hidden gastronomic resources of the region.
They don't know the secrets.

Let the easterners eat cheese in the park. After ten years of sushi and
chic, I find a plateful of perogies blanketed in fried onions very welcome. It
is only on the Prairies that I feel truly full. If there is truth to the old adage
that patriotism consists of the foods you ate as a child, then it is to the
Prairies that I owe my allegiance.

There is manna in the dustbowl.

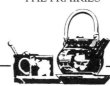

SUMMER SALAD WITH SUNFLOWER SEED DRESSING

Sunflower seeds salted in the shell are a most favoured snack on the Prairies, their popularity bolstered by the rumour that it takes more calories to get at the seed and eat it, than there are in the seeds. You can always find a bag on the dashboard of the car, or a few of them loose in purses and pockets. At summer resorts like Gimli and Winnipeg Beach, the summer residents spit seed shells and tell salty stories until their tongues are numb.

1	head leaf or Boston lettuce	1
1 cup	green beans, blanched	250 mL
12	cherry tomatoes	12
1 cup	snow peas, stems removed	250 mL
1 cup	bean sprouts	250 mL
4	green onions, chopped	4
½	head cauliflower, broken into florets	½
½ cup	unsalted sunflower seeds, shelled	125 mL
½ cup	grated old Cheddar cheese	125 mL
	Dressing:	
⅓ cup	sunflower seed oil	75 mL
⅓ cup	fresh lemon juice	75 mL
½ tsp	salt	2 mL
½ tsp	freshly ground pepper	2 mL

1. Break the lettuce into bite-sized pieces. Cut the green beans and tomatoes in half. Combine all the prepared vegetables in a large bowl.

2. To make the dressing, combine the sunflower seed oil, lemon juice, salt and pepper. Whisk briskly with a fork. Pour over the salad and toss.

3. Toss the dressed salad with the sunflower seeds and grated cheese.

Serves 8

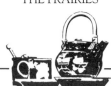

HOT BEET BORSCHT

The secret of good borscht lies in a rich stock flavoured with the perfect balance of sweet and sour. This is achieved by constant tasting and adjusting with lemon or brown sugar. When you're happy, serve the borscht with dark bread.

1 lb	boneless stewing beef, cut in 1-in/2.5-cm cubes	500 g
1 lb	short ribs	500 g
4	beets, scrubbed and unpeeled, with about 1 in/2.5 cm of the tops intact	4
2	medium onions, finely chopped	2
4	medium potatoes, quartered	4
1	28-oz/796-mL tin canned tomatoes	1
	Salt and freshly ground pepper to taste	
½ to ¾ cup	brown sugar	125 to 175 mL
3 to 4 Tbsp	lemon juice	50 to 75 mL

1. Place the meat, beets, onions, potatoes and tomatoes in a Dutch oven with enough water to cover. Bring to a boil. Turn down and simmer, uncovered, for 2 to 3 hours, or until the meat and vegetables are tender.

2. Remove the beets. Rinse under cold water and remove the skins. Slice and return to the soup. Add salt and pepper to taste.

3. Add brown sugar, then lemon juice to taste, adjusting quantities for the balance you like.

Serves 8

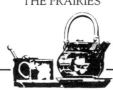

SMOKED CHICKEN PEKING STYLE

The style may be from Peking, but the recipe is from the Mandarin Restaurant in Winnipeg and can easily be made at home. You'll find the Szechuan peppercorns and star anise at oriental or specialty food stores. The chicken has a velvety texture and a gentle smoke flavour. This surprising method, which uses flour, sugar and black tea leaves, may also be used to smoke fish. You can also try it outdoors on a Coleman stove.

1 Tbsp	Szechuan peppercorns	15 mL
1 Tbsp	coarse salt	15 mL
1	2- to 3-lb/1- to 1.5-kg chicken, washed and patted dry	1
	Sesame oil	
	Master Sauce:	
1	green onion	1
3	slices fresh ginger	3
2	star anise	2
1	cinnamon stick	1
1 cup	soy sauce	250 mL
6 cups	chicken stock	1.5 L
¼ cup	granulated sugar	50 mL
1 Tbsp	dry sherry	15 mL
	Smoking Ingredients:	
2 Tbsp	white flour	25 mL
2 Tbsp	granulated sugar	25 mL
2 Tbsp	black tea leaves	25 mL

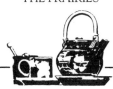

1. Stir-fry the peppercorns and salt in a small frying pan over low heat for about 5 minutes, or until the salt is light brown and the peppercorns are aromatic.

2. Rub the chicken with the salt-peppercorn mixture and marinate for 6 hours or overnight in the refrigerator.

3. Prepare the master sauce by combining all the sauce ingredients in a large pot. Boil vigorously for 10 minutes.

4. Add the chicken to the sauce, cover and cook for 7 minutes. Turn the chicken over and cook for another 7 minutes. Turn off the heat and let stand for 30 minutes. Remove the chicken to a platter to cool.

5. While the chicken is cooling, line a wok (or a large pot) and its cover with heavy-duty aluminum foil. Spread the smoking ingredients in the bottom of the wok. Prepare a rack in the wok by criss-crossing 4 wooden chopsticks to form a lattice (or you could use an oiled roasting rack). Place the chicken on the rack. Cover the wok with its cover.

6. Coil 2 wet tea towels around the seam. Cook over high heat until smoke comes out, then turn the heat to low. Smoke the chicken on each side for 5 minutes (remove the lid and turn the chicken near an open window if possible).

7. Remove the chicken from the wok and brush with sesame oil. When cool, cut into bite-sized pieces. Arrange on a platter and serve cold.

Serves 4 to 6

—*Y-Liang and Hu Wang, Mandarin Restaurant, Winnipeg, Manitoba*

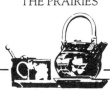

ROAST CAPON WITH BUCKWHEAT HONEY AND KASHA STUFFING

Buckwheat honey, a specialty of the Prairies, has its own smoky-rich flavour. Here it is spread on the poultry to produce a crisp, sweet skin. The bird is stuffed with dried apricots and kasha (bulgur), which is also very popular in Prairie households.

½ cup	buckwheat honey	125 mL
¼ cup	unsalted butter or rendered chicken fat	50 mL
½ tsp	salt	2 mL
1	capon, approximately 7 lb/3.5 kg	1
⅓ cup	sesame seeds	75 mL
	Stuffing:	
¼ cup	unsalted butter or rendered chicken fat	50 mL
2	medium onions, chopped	2
1½ cups	kasha (bulgur)	375 mL
2 cups	chicken stock	500 mL
⅓ cup	finely chopped dried apricots	75 mL
1 tsp	salt	5 mL
1 tsp	freshly ground pepper	5 mL

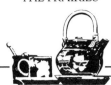

1. To make the stuffing, heat the butter over medium heat in a saucepan. Add the onions and cook for 5 minutes, or until the onion is translucent.

2. Add the kasha and cook for a further 5 minutes.

3. Stir in the chicken stock, dried apricots, salt and pepper. Bring to a boil, then reduce the heat to low, cover and cook for 5 minutes more. Remove from heat and let stand for 1 hour.

4. Preheat oven to 350°F/180°C.

5. In a small saucepan, heat the honey, butter and salt over low heat until the butter melts. Mix thoroughly.

6. Stuff the capon with the kasha-onion-apricot mixture.

7. Place the capon breast-side up in a large roasting pan, putting a little water in the bottom of the pan so the bird won't stick. Brush the capon thoroughly with the honey-butter mixture.

8. Roast the capon for 2 hours, brushing frequently with the honey-butter mixture and pan juices.

9. Remove the capon from the oven, brush it once more with the honey-butter mixture, and sprinkle it all over with the sesame seeds. Return to oven for 30 minutes more. Let stand 15 minutes before carving.

Serves 6

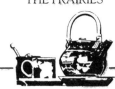

CABBAGE ROLLS

Cabbage rolls are, like borscht, based on a sweet and sour principle. The sweet is usually sugar (often brown); the sour is usually lemon juice. The combination of sweet and savoury is a common one in Russian and middle European cooking, and is often used, particularly in northern Canada, in fruit and game dishes.

In this recipe, prunes, raisins and apples provide some of the sweetness. To make the cabbage leaves flexible for rolling, freeze the entire head of cabbage a few days ahead of time, then let it thaw. The leaves will peel off easily.

1	head cabbage, separated into leaves	1
	Filling:	
1 lb	lean ground beef	500 g
2 cups	cooked brown rice	500 mL
½ cup	breadcrumbs	125 mL
1	egg	1
1 tsp	salt	5 mL
1 tsp	freshly ground pepper	5 mL
	Sauce:	
½ cup	tomato paste	125 mL
6	tomatoes, peeled or 1 28-oz/796-mL tin with liquid	6
1 cup	prunes, pitted	250 mL
½ cup	raisins	125 mL
3	apples, peeled and sliced	3
4	carrots, scraped and chopped	4
1 tsp	salt	5 mL
1 tsp	freshly ground pepper	5 mL
¼ cup	lemon juice	50 mL
2 Tbsp	brown sugar	25 mL

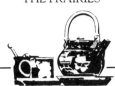

1. Prepare the filling by combining the ground beef, rice, breadcrumbs, egg, salt and pepper.

2. Roll about 1 Tbsp/15 mL of the meat mixture in each cabbage leaf, layering the cabbage rolls in a large casserole or baking dish as they are done.

3. To prepare the sauce, combine the tomato paste, fresh tomatoes with about 1 cup/250 mL water, or the tinned tomatoes, to make a loose sauce. Add the prunes, raisins, apples, carrots, salt and pepper.

4. Pour the sauce over the cabbage rolls. The sauce should cover the cabbage rolls. If it doesn't, add some water or more canned tomatoes.

5. Simmer the cabbage rolls very, very slowly over low heat on top of the stove. They will take nearly 4 hours to cook.

6. Halfway through the cooking, combine the lemon juice and brown sugar. Stir into the cabbage roll mixture, taking care not to break up the rolls. Taste for seasoning and add more lemon juice or sugar, or more salt or pepper if necessary.

7. Continue cooking for 2 hours.

Serves 6 to 8

POTATO AND CHEESE PEROGIES

Perogies are little pouches of dough. The most common filling is potato, or potato and cheese, but they can also be found filled with buckwheat or cabbage. Sometimes they are stuffed with meat and called veranekes or any number of other names given to them by the various groups that love them. They may be fried or boiled, served in a soup or on a plate with garlic sausage, fried onions and lots of sour cream.

1/4 cup	melted butter	50 mL
	Dough:	
2 cups	all-purpose flour	500 mL
1 tsp	salt	5 mL
1	egg	1
2/3 cup	cold water	150 mL
	Filling:	
1 cup	creamed cottage cheese	250 mL
2 cups	cooked and mashed potatoes	500 mL
1	green onion, finely chopped	1
1 tsp	finely chopped fresh dill	5 mL
	Salt and pepper to taste	

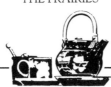

1. Grease a large Pyrex baking dish with the melted butter. Set aside.

2. To make the dough, sift the flour and salt into a small bowl.

3. Whisk the egg and water together. Mix into the flour. Knead the dough until smooth and shiny. Form into 2 balls. Cover with a damp tea towel and set aside.

4. To make the filling, place the cottage cheese in a sieve and hold under cold running tap water until the curds separate. Remove the excess water by tapping the sieve and allowing the curds to drain for a few minutes.

5. Mix the cottage cheese with the other filling ingredients.

6. Roll out the dough, 1 ball at a time, on a lightly floured surface to a thickness of $1/8$ in/3 mm or less (the thinner the better). Form a square approximately 14 in × 14 in/35 cm × 35 cm. Do not overwork the dough, or it will become less tender. Do not reroll odd pieces.

7. Cut the dough into 3-in/7.5-cm squares. Take each square in hand and stretch it slightly without making holes. Place 1 Tbsp/15 mL filling in the centre of each square and fold over to form a triangle, pinching the edges. Avoid getting any filling along the edges or they may not seal properly. Use a little flour if the dough becomes too moist from the filling.

8. Bring a large soup pot of water to a simmer. Place the filled perogies in the simmering water a few at a time. Do not crowd. Cook for a few minutes until they rise to the surface and look plumped out.

9. Remove the perogies to a colander. Drain well and then place them in the buttered dish, turning them to coat both sides with butter.

10. Preheat oven to 350°F/180°C. Bake the perogies, uncovered, for 10 to 15 minutes, or until plumped and slightly crisp on the bottom. Serve with sour cream, yogurt or fruit.

Makes 30 perogies

—*Judy Smith Comfort, Winnipeg, Manitoba*

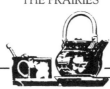

FRESHWATER WHITEFISH WITH WILD RICE STUFFING

This is a straightforward recipe that tastes best when the fish is at its freshest and the wild rice is prepared simply so that its nutty flavour comes through. Soaking the rice overnight is not necessary—instead, rinse the rice well and change the boiling water once.

1 cup	uncooked wild rice	250 mL
1	medium onion, chopped	1
2	stalks celery or 1 root (celeriac), chopped	2
1/3 cup	unsalted butter	75 mL
1 tsp	salt	5 mL
1 tsp	freshly ground pepper	5 mL
1 Tbsp	chopped parsley	15 mL
1/2 tsp	rosemary	2 mL
1	5-lb/2.5-kg whitefish, cleaned, head and tail on	1
1/2 cup	unsalted butter, melted	125 mL
1/2 tsp	salt	2 mL
1/2 tsp	freshly ground pepper	2 mL

1. To make the stuffing, rinse the rice thoroughly in a colander. Bring 2 qt/2 L water to a boil. Add the rice and boil for 20 minutes.

2. Drain the rice. Bring 2 qt/2 L fresh water to a boil. Add the rice and boil for 10 minutes more, or until the rice is tender but not mushy. Drain the rice and reserve.

3. Preheat oven to 500°F/260°C.

4. Cook the onion and celery in the 1/3 cup/75 mL butter until the onion is transparent.

5. Combine the onion and celery mixture with the boiled rice, salt, pepper, parsley and rosemary.

6. Stuff the mixture into the fish and secure the fish with wooden skewers or toothpicks.

7. Place the fish in a well-greased ovenproof pan. Pour the melted butter over the fish and sprinkle with salt and pepper.

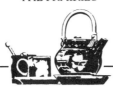

8. Bake for 15 minutes. Reduce the heat to 250°F/120°C and bake for a further 30 minutes, or until the fish flakes easily. Serve hot, with lemon slices.

Serves 4 to 6

MOM'S POPPY SEED COOKIES

Poppy seeds, so dark-blue in colour that they look black, are often used in middle and eastern European cooking, so pastries with them are common on the Prairies. These super cookies may be rolled and cut or squeezed from a press. Their secret is that some coconut is added, giving extra crunch and enhancing the nutty-sweetness of the poppy seeds.

3	eggs	3
scant 1 cup	granulated sugar	230 mL
¾ cup	vegetable oil	175 mL
3½ cups	all-purpose flour	875 mL
1 Tbsp	baking powder	15 mL
pinch	salt	pinch
¾ cup	poppy seeds	175 mL
¼ cup	unsweetened, dessicated coconut	50 mL

1. Preheat oven 375°F/190°C.

2. Beat the eggs until light. Gradually add the sugar and continue beating. Add the oil and beat for a further 2 minutes.

3. Sift together the flour, baking powder and salt. Add all at once to the egg mixture, mixing it in thoroughly.

4. Fold in the poppy seeds and the coconut. At this point, the batter should not be too sticky. If it is, add up to ½ cup/125 mL more flour until it can be rolled.

5. On a floured board, roll out the dough about ⅓ in/1 cm thick. Cut into desired shapes with a cookie cutter. Lay on ungreased cookie sheets and bake for 10 minutes, or until the cookies are a light golden brown.

Makes 30 to 40 cookies

—Ada Berney, Winnipeg, Manitoba

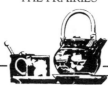

HUGE CINNAMON ROLLS

You can slice them and toast them and share them with your cousin, but a real Prairie eater will eat a whole roll with lots of butter.

1 1/2 cups	milk	375 mL
1/4 cup	granulated sugar	50 mL
2 tsp	salt	10 mL
1/4 cup	unsalted butter	50 mL
1 tsp	granulated sugar	5 mL
1/2 cup	lukewarm water	125 mL
1 Tbsp	active dry yeast	15 mL
1	egg, well beaten	1
5 1/2 to 6 cups	all-purpose flour	1.4 to 1.5 L
3/4 cup	unsalted butter, melted	175 mL
1 1/2 cups	brown sugar	375 mL
1 Tbsp	cinnamon	15 mL
1/2 cup	raisins	125 mL
1/2 cup	walnut pieces	125 mL

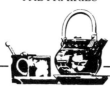

1. Scald the milk by heating it to just below the boiling point. Add ¼ cup/ 50 mL granulated sugar, salt and ¼ cup/50 mL butter. Stir until the butter melts. Cool to lukewarm.

2. Meanwhile, dissolve 1 tsp/5 mL granulated sugar in the lukewarm water, sprinkle yeast over the mixture and let it stand for 10 minutes. Stir with a fork.

3. Mix together the milk mixture, softened yeast and beaten egg.

4. Beat in 3 cups/750 mL flour. Then add the remaining flour until the dough is of a consistency to knead. Knead until smooth and elastic.

5. Place the dough in a buttered bowl. Cover with a tea towel and let rise in a warm place until doubled in bulk, about 1½ hours.

6. Punch down the dough and turn it onto a lightly buttered board. Roll into a rectangle 14 in × 20 in/35 cm × 50 cm. Brush with ½ cup/125 mL melted butter.

7. Mix together 1 cup/250 mL brown sugar with the cinnamon. Sprinkle evenly over the dough. Sprinkle with raisins and walnuts.

8. Starting from the longer side, roll the dough like a jellyroll and pinch to seal edges. Cut the roll into 12 thick slices.

9. Combine ¼ cup/50 mL melted butter and ½ cup/125 mL brown sugar and spread on the bottom of a jellyroll pan or cookie sheet (you may need more than one sheet to accommodate the buns). Place each bun cut-side down in the prepared pans, leaving room for them to expand.

10. Cover the rolls with a tea towel and let them rise in a warm place until doubled in bulk, about 45 minutes.

11. Preheat oven to 375°F/190°C. Bake rolls for 25 to 30 minutes. Invert at once onto serving plates and serve warm with butter.

Makes 12 large rolls

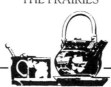

FLAPPER PIE

You don't see that much of this heaping custard-meringue pie anymore. It was a specialty of the Salisbury House chain and part of life for anyone who ate their wonderful nips and ended an already heavy meal with its three layers of Graham cracker crust, custard filling and meringue topping. This recipe is from a truck stop restaurant on the outskirts of Calgary.

	Crust:	
1 ½ cups	Graham wafer crumbs	375 mL
⅓ cup	brown sugar	75 mL
¼ cup	melted butter	50 mL
	Custard:	
6	egg yolks	6
½ cup	granulated sugar	125 mL
¼ cup	cornstarch	50 mL
4 cups	whole milk	1 L
2 tsp	vanilla extract	10 mL
	Meringue:	
6	egg whites	6
¼ cup	granulated sugar	50 mL
½ tsp	cornstarch	2 mL
1 Tbsp	Graham wafer crumbs	15 mL

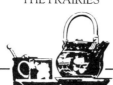

1. Preheat oven to 350°F/180°C.

2. To make the crust, combine the Graham wafer crumbs, brown sugar and melted butter. Press into a 10-in/2-L pie plate. Bake for 10 minutes. Set aside.

3. To make the custard, beat the egg yolks slightly with a fork. Add the granulated sugar and cornstarch.

4. Heat the milk to just below the boiling point and slowly add it to egg-sugar mixture, stirring constantly. Cook over low heat, stirring constantly, until thickened. Add the vanilla extract. Cool.

5. To make the meringue, beat the egg whites until soft peaks form. Add the granulated sugar and cornstarch and continue beating until the peaks stiffen.

6. Pour the cooled custard filling into the pie crust. Spoon the meringue on top of the custard.

7. Sprinkle 1 Tbsp/15 mL Graham wafer crumbs over the meringue. Bake the pie for about 15 minutes, until the top is golden brown. Chill for several hours before serving.

Serves 6

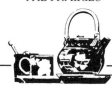

CHOCOLATE MOUSSE CAKE

There are purists who argue that cheesecake should only be white and chocolate mousse should only be chocolate. My Auntie Carole combines both to reach new heights in richness and dense chocolate flavour. This is a wonderful dessert that also freezes well.

	Crust:	
⅓ cup	melted butter	75 mL
25 to 30	chocolate wafers, crushed	25 to 30
	Filling:	
2 cups	cream cheese	500 mL
1 cup	granulated sugar	250 mL
4	eggs, separated	4
2 tsp	vanilla	10 mL
12 oz	chocolate chips, melted	350 g
1 cup	whipping cream	250 mL

1. Preheat oven to 325°F/160°C.

2. To make the crust, add the melted butter to the crushed wafers and press into the bottom of a 10-in/4.5-L spring-form pan. Bake for 10 minutes.

3. Blend the cream cheese and ½ cup/125 mL sugar together. Add the egg yolks, vanilla and melted chocolate chips and blend in.

4. In a separate bowl, beat the egg whites until soft peaks form. Gradually add the remaining sugar. Fold the sweetened egg whites into the chocolate-cream cheese mixture.

5. Pour the filling into the spring-form pan, smoothing it on top of the baked chocolate crust. Refrigerate.

6. Just before serving, whip the cream and spread it over the cake.

Serves 10 to 12

—*Carole Berney, Winnipeg, Manitoba*

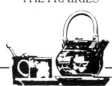

WINNIPEG CHEESECAKE

This cake once won top honours in a cheesecake contest in Winnipeg, considered by some to be the cheesecake capital of Canada. Wherever you are, use the creamiest cream cheese you can find (use People's Co-operative cream cheese if you live in Manitoba).

³/₄ cup	Graham wafer crumbs	175 mL
¹/₃ cup	brown sugar	75 mL
	Peel of 1 lemon, grated	
¹/₄ tsp	cardamom	1 mL
¹/₃ cup	melted butter	75 mL
2 lb	cream cheese	1 kg
4	eggs	4
³/₄ cup	granulated sugar	175 mL
	Juice from ¹/₂ lemon	
1 tsp	vanilla	5 mL

1. Preheat oven to 350°F/180°C.
2. To make the crust, combine the first 5 ingredients and mix thoroughly. Press into the bottom of a buttered 10-in/4.5-L springform pan.
3. In a large bowl, combine the cream cheese, eggs, granulated sugar, lemon juice and vanilla. Beat thoroughly and pour on top of the crust.

4. Bake for 35 minutes.
5. When the baking is done, turn off the oven, prop the oven door open with a folded tea towel and let the cake stand in the oven for about 1 hour. Refrigerate for several hours before serving.

Serves 10 to 12

—Heather Cram, Winnipeg, Manitoba

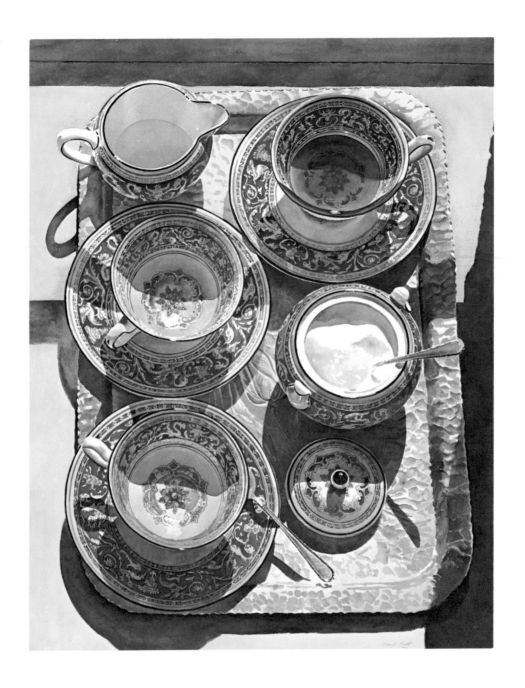

Tea tray with Florentine

*I have always loved the look of sugar in a china
sugar bowl. That little mound of tiny crystals—
partly lit by the sun coming through the thin china
and partly lit by the sun coming through the nearest
window. (M.P.)*

BRITISH COLUMBIA

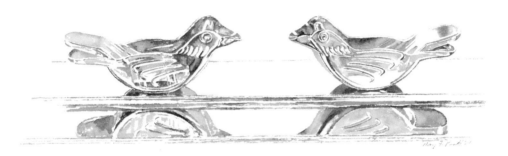

In British Columbia, food has as much entertainment value as it has nutritional. I once spoke to a man who roasted a sirloin of beef on the manifold of his '51 Packard on the way to a picnic on Vancouver Island. When he reached his destination, he unpacked a stick of French bread and a bottle of red wine and had hot beef sandwiches. Writer Eve Rockett has been driving around Vancouver for years in a Volkswagen van with the name "Van Ordinaire '68" painted on its side. And only in British Columbia could they hold a dog food eating contest where twenty people signed up, but only twelve showed.

It's easy to be silly about food in British Columbia. Unlike the rest of Canada where the regional cuisine has developed in spite of the climate and scarcity, British Columbia has always been comfortable in its bounty—so comfortable that people have the luxury of an almost playful attitude toward food. Wonderful food, along with all the other amenities like warmth, sea breezes and roses, has come easily to British Columbia. The only challenge to the development of a unique cuisine has been how to coax the natives off their yoga mats to go and collect it.

This has been a bitter pill for the rest of us to swallow, but we have made it go down more easily with unkind jokes about granola and alfalfa sprouts. "My impression of B.C. food," revealed a woman from Ontario, shivering at the time in Toronto over a cup of lukewarm tea, "is that they eat salmon in the spring and lotus the rest of the year—except in Victoria, where they eat scones."

They also eat the best crab in the world, superb Japanese and Chinese food, and some of the best chocolate in Canada. They have farmlands that bulge with fresh fruits and Oriental vegetables, waters that jump with shrimp, prawns, oysters and the makings of the most luxurious bouillabaisse ever. What's more, this is the province that includes the price of a massage on its medical plan.

In fact, the appreciation of this largesse is fairly recent. British Columbians have confided that until the sixties, people cooked from cans and ate white bread just like everyone else. There were few restaurants in the cities, and those few were dull. Like other large Canadian cities of those years, Vancouver and Victoria limped along with the odd luxury steak house, and the best eating was to be found in private homes, private clubs and in the dining rooms of large hotels. But even in those sheltered spots, fresh fish was exotic and crunchy vegetables were suspect.

The change, when it came, was quite dramatic. Settlements of what were sneeringly referred to as "granolas" helped, with their interest in going back to the land. The land was easy to go back to—soil was generous, the growing period was long and you didn't have to freeze while you collected the food. The fashion for freshness that swept North America in the seventies caught on quickly in British Columbia. It was easy to reject packaged foods and heavy meat meals, considering the alternatives available.

The new emphasis on health and fitness was strong in a place where everyone felt so good anyway. I once watched an elderly woman enjoy a sherbet in a downtown ice cream parlour. She sat at a tiny table by herself, surrounded by shopping bags, her knees akimbo. She wore no makeup and there was nothing about the way she adorned herself to suggest her passionate commitment to her afternoon treat.

But she ate her mandarin sherbet cup with a joy that was palpable. She would scoop the bright orange sherbet from around the edges of the cup, taste the tip of each spoonful, then lick it until the tiny silver utensil was shining clean. In this manner she scraped the last of the sweetness from the inside of the cup. When she rose to pay her bill, I ran after her. "Do you come here often?"

She grinned a big orange smile. "Usually I just have a cup of tea. But I saw this new place and came in for the sherbet because I thought I needed the vitamins. And, d'ya know? That sherbet must be full of health. I got a real lift from it."

In its culinary trends, British Columbia is influenced far more by California than by Quebec or Ontario. Orange sherbet replaced a coffee and Danish there long before it did anywhere else. Salads and sprouts were commonplace in Vancouver when Toronto was still looking at a plate of alfalfa sprouts as if it were a back-combed hairpiece. There are dishes on the menus of sunny outdoor restaurants that are as baffling for an eastern Canadian to understand as they are to eat. Messy Muffuletta on Focaccia Bread with Wine Salami turned out to be a cheese and sausage sandwich on crusty bread that completely fell apart at first bite, leaving a delicious mess to be licked up from forearms and fingers.

But the most influential factor in the burst of healthy eating that has taken place throughout the province has been immigration, especially of Orientals, whose cuisine lent itself to B.C.'s natural endowments.

Oriental cookery emphasizes freshness and the minimal processing of quality produce. Seafood is treated gently, cooked just until the rawness is gone so that the flavour is kept. Fresh fish is steamed, its meat left moist; fresh vegetables are quickly seared with heat, their crunch sealed.

The history of the acceptance of Orientals in western Canada has been repressive, but in general, Oriental cuisine has been welcomed whole-heartedly. A government-sponsored pamphlet for restaurant kitchens is printed in the two official languages of British Columbia's culinary community: English and Chinese.

But occasionally there are still cultural clashes. A few years ago there was an uproar in Vancouver about the ducks dripping in the windows of Chinese restaurants and grocery stores. By tradition, the ducks are barbecued, then left to drip in the open air until the fat leaves the body, the meat becomes moist and the skin turns crisp and reddish-brown. The duck is hacked into pieces when it is sold; it is wonderful dipped into fiery hot mustards and plum sauces, or wrapped in Mandarin pancakes with some stir-fried noodles and sprouts. To the Chinese, who for years let the ducks hang in windows to seduce hungry passersby into the store, the method was acceptable and appealing. To the germ-phobic Caucasians who argued that the ducks had been foisted upon them, the method was unsanitary at best. Attempts were made to forbid the practice. But they were fought, and eventually the ducks—and tradition—won out.

One of the more obvious benefits of the Oriental influence is the way Oriental eateries have made diners aware of local seafood specialties such as the Dungeness crab. Fished all along the coast, this shellfish was once served mainly at private parties on Vancouver Island. The crabs were not easily available in street markets or in restaurants. Now in Vancouver there is hardly a Chinese restaurant worth its soya that doesn't have a crab tank.

The Dungeness crab, named for the town of Dungeness in Washington,

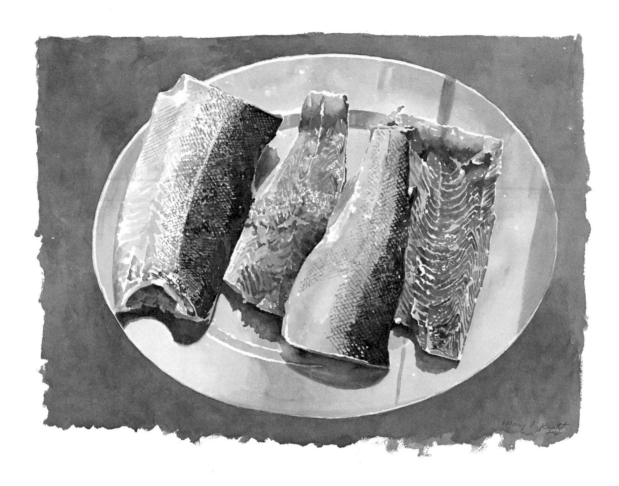

Salmon on a Rosenthal platter

The perfection of design in fish is quite lovely and absolutely functional. The black back is difficult for predators from above to discern in black water, the belly is silver so that underwater predators think they're looking at the sky. Filleted, lying glistening on an oval porcelain plate outdoors on the grass beside a brook, the sight was just like early summer. (M.P.)

is one I would always choose over the snow crab or even the gargantuan Alaska king crab, which gives its legs to so many Canadian restaurants. The Dungeness is a large crab and its meat is sweet and firm. It is best eaten at its simplest, when it has been pulled fresh from the water and quickly steamed.

It takes a long time to eat a crab. Most of the meat is in the legs, but there is also some in the muscle that joins the leg to the body, and there is more in tender shards between pieces of cartilage, if you have the patience to search. When crab is done in the black bean and garlic sauce most common in Vancouver's Chinatown, a whole crab is sautéed and simmered in what looks like chunky and shiny black mud. You still have to eat the things with your hands, since there exists no instrument outside of a surgical theatre designed for separating the hard shell from the soft flesh. You have to edit the dish, scraping off the black bean sauce first, cracking the crab, then running the white meat through the sauce you've hoarded at the side of your plate.

There's more than seafood to Vancouver's Chinatown. The markets along Pender Street carry fresh water chestnuts, fresh lichee nuts (which are a completely different food from the sticky-sweet ones sold in tins and served to Occidentals who insist that a Chinese meal must end with dessert). There are fresh bamboo shoots and many other Chinese vegetables and flavourings. At Yang's on Main Street every Saturday at noon there is a wonderful show of fresh noodle-making by the chef. There's showmanship in other Oriental places, too. One sushi bar serves the colourful little pieces by conveyor belt. The chef behind the counter makes them, puts them on the belt and sends them around the track. Customers pick out the ones they want as the sushi goes on by.

One can hardly think of British Columbia without thinking of salmon. I find it completely different in texture and taste from the Atlantic salmon, but no less wonderful.

It is a measure of our technological times that Canadians can freely argue the merits of the rich west coast salmon over the juicy, lighter meat of the East. Fresh salmon is as available in Winnipeg as it is in Toronto, although it is usually B.C. salmon that is more readily found. But it is expensive. According to Michelle Daignault of the federal Department of Fisheries and Oceans, the reason for the cost is that everyone everywhere likes salmon. "Foreign markets such as Sweden, Italy and Japan are willing to pay high prices for Canadian salmon. That means we have to pay high prices, too."

We do. In 1982 Canadians bought five thousand tons of fresh and frozen

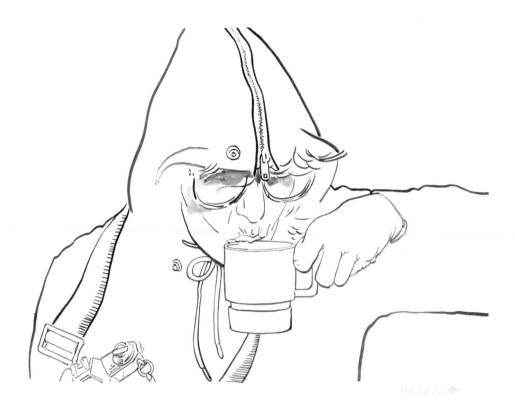

Linda with cocoa

salmon. We like salmon better than any other fish. Some of us don't even think of it as fish. People who normally don't order fish in a restaurant will often order a grilled salmon steak, paying as much as they once did for New York strip.

If salmon is to be our steak of the eighties, we ought to treat it with the respect it deserves. Fresh salmon has endured awful insults in the name of culinary fashion. It has been puréed to a pulp and creamed to a paste. I've seen it cowering in crêpes and gasping for breath under thick sauces. Priced as high as filet mignon, it deserves as simple and proud a delivery. For purists there are only two ways to eat it—hot with hollandaise or cold with mayonnaise—and only two ways to cook it—poached so gently that it flakes at the touch of a fork or grilled over an open flame so that its edges become crispy with butter and charred fish juices. If the fish is to be eaten hot, I'm partial to the open flame, particularly if the salmon is flamed over mesquite charcoal (made from the mesquite bush that grows in the southern United States).

The mating of fish to flame is nothing new. Indians traditionally cooked a whole salmon on top of a tepee-shaped holder made with sticks and string. The tepee cooking rack was then set over a wood fire. In Atlantic Canada, the Micmac Indians butterflied a whole salmon and spread it skin side down on a hardwood board and faced it to an open fire. The tethered fish faced the flame for as long as three hours, long enough for the juices to flow from the fish, be collected and brushed back on.

Enterprising salmon grillers in British Columbia have found modern ways to update the native theme. David Winestock in Victoria follows a method still used by local natives. He marinates salmon fillets in water, brown sugar and salt for two hours. The he heats hardwood chips in his barbecue under a closed cover. Just before dinner, he lays the marinated fish fillets in an open baking dish, places them inside the barbecue and lets the smoking hardwood cook the fish. It is fabulous. Pat Todd, a Vancouver executive, barbecues salmon inside the family fireplace using an old-fashioned toaster rack to secure the fillets. He bastes them with lemon juice and butter for flavour and to prevent dryness. Because fresh salmon can be so easily cubed and skewered, I make shishkabobs, alternating cubes of salmon with pieces of cucumber and basting them with butter-oil and lemon juice while they're on the flame.

Whole salmon is best poached. Lay the fish in a poacher or in any covered pan large enough to contain it and fill the container with some liquid until three-quarters of the fish is submerged. The most popular liquids are fish stock or court bouillon, a mixture of white wine and water, or sometimes even milk with fresh herbs such as dill or tarragon. I'm partial to using cider, especially the delicious apple or pear ciders that are being produced in British Columbia. (Keep a little of the cider aside to sip while the salmon is cooking. With a squirt of fresh lime juice, it is a terrific drink.)

Brave souls who somehow have the nerve to risk a fifty-dollar fish have developed a wonderful method for poaching salmon in a dishwasher. You must have a dishwasher with a drying cycle, because the new ones with energy-saving features don't give off enough heat. Wash and pat dry a five-pound salmon and stuff it with fresh parsley, dill, lemon or any fresh herbs you like. Sprinkle the outside with salt and freshly ground pepper. Wrap the fish in two layers of foil—no less or you'll have fish juice in your cutlery tray, and no more or the heat won't penetrate. Then fit the salmon onto the middle of the top rack of the dishwasher. Run the machine for two complete cycles without peeking. When the fish is done, it will look and taste moister than it does when it is cooked conventionally (this is the main advantage of this offbeat method; although salmon is a fairly fat fish, it slips easily into dryness). Serve the fish hot or cold with mayonnaise, hollandaise or melted lemon butter.

Smoked B.C. salmon also shouldn't be missed. There is an inclination to gussy it up—to wrap it around cream cheese. I was once so appalled at a menu offering of smoked salmon wrapped around a fresh fig and drizzled with vinaigrette, that I ordered it. But the only thing smoked salmon should be twirled around before it's eaten is a bare finger.

I was introduced to the chocolate of British Columbia when I lived in Winnipeg and my cousin Lorraine would bring back the superb pastries from the Notte's Bon Ton Pastry and Confectionary in Vancouver. The pastries were tiny, delicate treasures of chocolate surrounding cream fillings that weren't too sweet or marzipan that had the flavour of real almonds. That chocolate is still as good as the first batch the Notte family made when they started in 1928.

I like to make a meal of the Bon Ton pastries when I go there now. I still like the chocolate rolls with the pink and white centres, but I've also done very well with those filled only with chocolate cream. I spent an afternoon touring through Vancouver's chocolate outlets not long ago, beginning the trip at the Bon Ton, then continuing through several glittery shops that sold hand-dipped chocolates filled with soft fresh cream that was gently flavoured with various fruits or even more chocolate.

It's hard to stop eating when you're faced with chocolate that good, and British Columbia is not the place to try to stop eating chocolate. Vancouver and Victoria are smeared with chocolate stores that sell the pretty boxed confections sought by tourists from Britain and the United States. There are Roger's Victoria creams, which are famous all over, and Purdy's marzipan bars—slender columns of chocolate enrobing textured marzipan. Those familiar with Purdy's sample trays know that the code question, "What do you have to offer today?" will signal to the saleslady that it's okay to bring out the samples. This practice is common to many stores selling candy and baked goods. They understand the lure of sweets, of the song that sweet things sing to the seducible. One taste and you might buy the shop.

There are so many chocolate outlets in Vancouver that the Yellow Pages has devoted an entire section to them. Sometimes you can also find seconds of moulded chocolates: chocolate Easter bunnies with only one ear, or a Santa Claus with a chipped toy bag. Vancouver also has an annual chocolate festival, where local chocolate makers display their wares for the public. As Erwin Dobeli of the William Tell restaurant in Vancouver says: "I wouldn't dare put out a dessert menu without chocolate on it. It's the most demanded flavour here."

British Columbia's chocolate is famous in part because of the tourists who buy it. B.C. attracts a lot of tourists, especially Americans who flock to Victoria, a city that makes the most of its colonial ties.

Victoria is as British as you can get outside of Brighton, a fact reinforced by the double-decker buses and white-gloved ladies who take tea in the many tea shops that dot the area. Though the cakes and sandwiches are much the same as you'd have in England, in Canada the food is often served in amounts that would put the average English person, used to a little snack at four, under the table. While most of the tea shops serve the traditional cream tea which includes scones, cream (Devon clotted, if possible, but more likely stiffly whipped cream), sandwiches and cakes, in Canadian shops the scones are huge, the sandwiches are thick and the slices of cake are mammoth.

The most famous tea in all of Canada used to be the one at the majestic Empress Hotel in Victoria, but even that has succumbed to North American efficiency. Gone are the dowagers in wing chairs sipping tea in translucent china cups. They have been replaced by scores of plaid-shirted tourists standing in line with their numbered cards awaiting metal carts clattering with heavy glass dishes. The pastry and sandwiches are all there, but so is Jello.

With the appreciation of pastry and chocolate in British Columbia, it is no accident that another of British Columbia's best-known confections is two layers of chocolate separated by a layer of white icing. The Nanaimo Bar, a cookie so sweet that it makes your ears ring, is said to come from Nanaimo, a legend to which the Nanaimo Chamber of Commerce clings with some tenacity, though there is constant controversy over the origin of this famous cookie. Averill Winestock of Victoria, whose plan it is one day to open a pub in Nanaimo and call it the Nanaimo Bar, knew them as a child as Auntie Reenie Bars. I have heard them called Saskatoon Bars and New York Bars. Whatever their name, they are eaten everywhere in Canada, including in St. John's, Newfoundland, where I once saw them advertised in a restaurant as Nameeno (sic) Bars.

Nanaimo has other things to boast about. Mountain squab, young fledgling pigeons, are raised on farms near Nanaimo. Properly cooked, squab has the consistency of tender steak, but its flavour is richer than chicken. Like most foods with rich flavour, it calls for simple preparation. I like to brown the birds quickly in butter, then sprinkle them with salt, pepper, garlic and onions. I add a bit of red wine for liquid, then simmer them slowly on the stove for about 40 minutes.

Squab was wonderfully received in 1983, when a Canadian team of

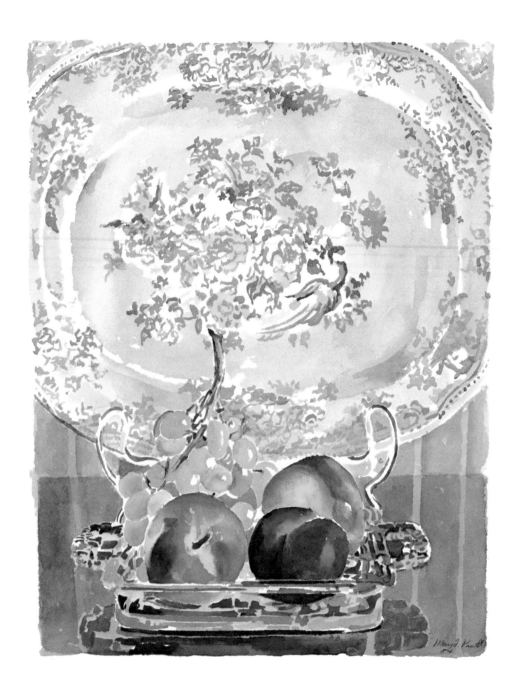

Blue pheasant platter and fruit

*We can't harvest fruit like this in Newfoundland so I
have never seen a peach actually growing. I consider
them so precious that when I buy them I seldom eat
them—I just like to look at them. (M.P.)*

chefs took 240 Vancouver Island squab to Japan for an international gourmet fair and returned with five gold medals. It is less well received here, perhaps because of its size and because people are never sure how to eat it. The main rule, according to an American fashion editor whose subspecialty is eating etiquette, is "never pick up the body with your hands."

There is no problem eating many of British Columbia's other specialties with your hands. The Okanagan Valley is the source of much fresh produce that is consumed throughout Canada—especially apples and peaches. But there are also crops you wouldn't think of, such as the hazelnuts that Hazel and John Spencer raise in Rosedale.

Fresh nuts are a treat for anyone who always thought that nuts grew in cellophane packages, and John Spencer has made his name in nuts by devising a new method for harvesting them. In the fall, when the nuts are mature, he sends helicopters to hover just above the trees. The force from the whirling blades shakes the trees so traumatically that they release their nuts. The fallen nuts are then easily gathered. This method has quite revolutionized the harvest. Until then, harvesters would have to shake the branches from the ground until the nuts fell off—a laborious and time-consuming procedure.

Exciting as Spencer's new process is, it happens only once a year, thus leaving Hazel and John with lots of time on their hands. They use some of that time to devise jokes to one-up all the puns people make on their life at the nut farm. Spencer has a calling card with a few of the best of them. "First to Blow My Nuts Off by Helicopter" it says on one corner of the card. "First to Have My Nuts on Television" it boasts on another, topping them both with his ultimate brag: "First to Put My Nuts in a 50 lb Bag and Fill It."

Another thing the Spencers do with their nuts is make them into delicious cakes. Here is their easy recipe for hazelnut cake. Beat 3 eggs and add 2/3 cup/150 mL sugar. Continue beating until the mixture becomes quite thick. Blend in 1 1/2 cups/375 mL ground hazelnuts. Bake in a 9-in/ 2-L square buttered baking pan in a 325°F/160°C oven for 1 hour, or until the cake is golden and springy to the touch.

If you want lots of food, there is no better place to get it than in the construction camps in British Columbia. Food is pretty important to these guys who have nothing much to do but work and eat, isolated as they are from other distractions. The workers will tell you that until they protested, the camp food was pretty awful. There was lots of it, but it was boring, consisting of things like baked beans on toast and fatty stews. Now the unions make sure that the meals their members get keep them happy. I'd heard tales of such meals: how European-trained chefs slaved for hours in steaming camp kitchens to please the hearty hungers of men who spent hours at gruelling outdoor labours. The food is more than fuel; it has to be of sufficient quantity and quality to provide diversion and pleasure. "It also has to be good enough," added one chef, "so that the guys don't throw it back at you."

It wasn't easy to coax a lunch from the director of one of these camps. "You don't need to come here to see how well these guys eat," he said. "Take my word for it. We spoil them rotten seven days a week. These guys are so fussy, the next thing they'll want is breakfast in bed."

I settled for lunch at the table. But on two conditions: I was not to mention the name or location of the camp and I was not to sit with the men at lunch. ("Those guys hate having women in the kitchen and I hate having trouble with the union.").

The camp was somewhere in the wilds of Vancouver Island and the dining hall was in the midst of a number of sturdy but makeshift buildings. I thought it was all quite austere, until I saw the food: huge cauldrons steaming with freshly made clam chowder; a high-hatted chef chopping mounds of fresh parsley for garnish; silver trays of fresh cod glistening white under dollops of butter—the fish had been caught locally and rushed to the camp that morning. Elsewhere there were oceans of Swedish meatballs reclining in a rich cream sauce with noodles waiting at their side. A joint of rare roast beef and another of pork were steaming in stainless-steel ovens. Fresh bread was being kept warm. The bread was made by the other chef whose specialty was baking. That day for lunch he had also prepared blueberry and lemon pies, chocolate cake, blueberry and coconut squares and some custards. And there were twelve flavours of ice cream in the freezer.

For a first course there were mountains of chipped ice that held hills of pink shrimp, forests of Greek salad (the real McCoy—with Feta cheese and salty black olives). There was marinated herring and trays of various cheeses cut into triangles and laid out like fallen dominoes. There were platters of thinly sliced rare roast beef and turkey breast. I could go on, but you get the idea.

The doors to the dining room opened to admit the men at 11:50. They walked in single file to the food, filled their plates, ate without conversation or comment and had cleared the dining room twenty minutes later.

Later I asked the director if I might take a picture of the dining room and some of the men.

"Not a chance."

"Were some of those big tough guys camera shy?" I wondered.

"Camera shy!" he hooted. "Hell, they're wanted!"

The grand feasting at the construction camps is not the only well-kept secret in B.C. I've found that you have to coax the names of offbeat restaurants from the locals. Ask them for the names of the best places to eat and they're likely to name the spiffy Pavillon in the Four Seasons Hotel, or Barbara Gordon's La Cachette or one of Umberto's Menghi's posh Italian places. Columnist Denny Boyd of the Vancouver *Sun* says that Vancouverites tell visitors, especially visitors from the East, about the luxury restaurants and save the finds for themselves: "We'll tell you about Le Pavillon, but we'll eat at Bud's" (Bud's Halibut on Denman, which Boyd says has the best cole slaw in the West, a claim challenged by those who have dined at the Ukee Bowling Alley in Port Alberni). There's also The Only for seafood, where the stuff is cheap and fast and good, and any number of smaller seafood places, like the ones that serve oyster burgers down at the Campbell Street docks.

Some of Canada's greatest restaurant success stories began in British Columbia. The Keg began there in the sixties, endearing itself to the free-roaming youth who loved the place for their cheap hits of Grand Marnier. I've watched more Grand Marnier being drunk in British Columbia than anywhere else in Canada. Certainly everyone I have ever known from B.C. drinks it, though, unlike their Calgary neighbours, they drink it after meals, rather than before or instead of meals. The Old Spaghetti Factory, now an enormously popular chain with locations throughout the world, began in Vancouver, the inspiration of psychologist Lee Paulos, who understood well the compelling effect of serving a $2 meal in a $10 atmosphere.

The first hint that anyone on the outside had about what was really going on in British Columbia's food scene was in 1980 at the International Culinary Olympics in Frankfurt, Germany. Held every four years, the culinary games are the place where nations compete for medals, only at the Culinary Olympics they compete with menus, not muscles. British Columbia had been entirely left out of the national Canadian team. They had auditioned, but had been eliminated. Angry, four of B.C.'s more persistent chefs found funding and took their skills, along with heaping cargoes of salmon, scallops and shrimp, to Germany. The British Columbia team won gold medals in their division, while the Canadian team placed only third in theirs.

One of the B.C. chefs, Bruno Marti, was triumphant: "We knew we weren't just steak and potato eaters anymore. Now we've proven that B.C.

can do food as good as anywhere in Canada." Four years later, Marti led the Canadian team to world victory at the 1984 Culinary Olympics.

His confidence was confirmed when the International Wine and Food Society, a group based in London, England, chose Vancouver for its 1983 international convention. Hobby eaters from all over the world came to eat B.C. lamb cradled in pastry, scallops fished off B.C. shores and Pacific baby shrimps.

It has been a while now since Vancouver limped along with a few luxury steak houses and the best food was found in the hotel dining rooms and in people's private homes. And it has been years since the bounty from the ocean and the array of produce was barely given lip service. These days B.C. has everything from granola to gourmet. Considering the province's climate, it seems inequitable that British Columbians have wonderful food, too.

Life must be swell in a province where, when they are hungry, all they have to do is go out into the garden and eat roses.

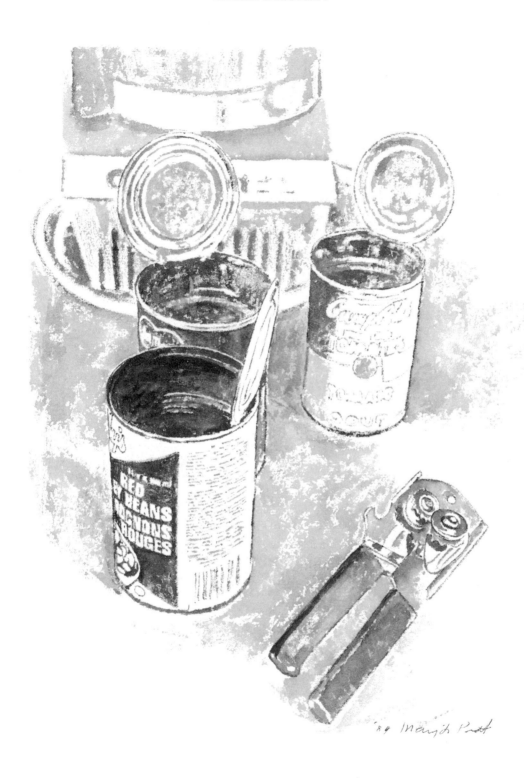

Cans and can opener

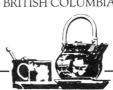

SPINACH, ORANGE AND MANGO SALAD

Pretty salads that combine fruit and leaf have become popular all along the west coast, their sunny tastes a reflection of California warmth.

The tart dressing is a perfect foil for the sweet, juicy fruit in this recipe. Soft, ripe honeydew or cantaloupe may be substituted for the mango. Do not refrigerate the salad, since room temperatures will bring out the best flavour. Instead, serve the salad on chilled plates.

1 lb	spinach	500 g
2	oranges	2
1	grapefruit	1
2	mangoes	2
1 Tbsp	grated onion	15 mL
½ tsp	salt	2 mL
½ tsp	freshly ground pepper	2 mL
1 Tbsp	Dijon mustard	15 mL
2 Tbsp	white wine vinegar	25 mL
1 tsp	fresh lemon juice	5 mL
⅔ cup	olive oil	150 mL

1. Wash and thoroughly dry the spinach. Remove the stems and discard them.

2. Peel and section the oranges and grapefruit.

3. Peel the mangoes and remove the pits. Cut the mangoes into strips.

4. Prepare the dressing by combining the onion, salt, pepper, mustard, vinegar and lemon juice in a small bowl. Mix well.

5. Beat the olive oil into the dressing very slowly. Continue beating until the mixture thickens.

6. Combine the spinach and fruit in a chilled salad bowl. Pour on the dressing and toss gently but thoroughly. Let stand for 10 minutes. Serve on chilled plates.

Serves 4 to 6

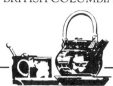

FETTUCCINE WITH PROSCIUTTO AND PEAS

Pasta was booming in B.C. long before it became fashionable in eastern Canada, largely because of Umberto Menghi, who operates a number of Italian restaurants in Vancouver. This easily prepared pasta dish becomes a meal with a salad and dry white wine. Prosciutto, the lightly smoked Italian ham, is available in specialty stores. Each slice should be paper thin; avoid any that looks dry at the edges. Also, use freshly grated Parmesan cheese—preferably Parmigiano Reggiano, if you're feeling flush.

1 lb	fettuccine noodles	500 g
6	slices prosciutto ham	6
2 Tbsp	butter	25 mL
1½ cups	peas, fresh or thawed	375 mL
1 tsp	white pepper	5 mL
¾ cup	light cream	175 mL
1 cup	freshly grated Parmesan cheese	250 mL

1. Cook the fettuccine in rapidly boiling salted water. Fresh homemade pasta will take only 1 or 2 minutes; store-bought pasta will take 3 or 4 minutes and dry packaged pasta will take about 5 to 7 minutes. Cook the pasta *al dente*, or just tender to the bite.

2. While the pasta is cooking, cut the prosciutto into wide strips and cook it in the butter until the ham is just soft but not crisp.

3. Add the peas and cook until they are tender but not mushy. Add the white pepper but avoid the temptation to add salt (the ham and Parmesan cheese are usually salty enough).

4. Drain the fettuccine and add it to the saucepan with the prosciutto and peas.

5. Add the cream and cook for 1 minute, or just until the cream is hot and begins to thicken.

6. Add the freshly grated Parmesan and toss to mix. Serve immediately with extra cheese.

Serves 4 as a main course or 6 as an appetizer

—Umberto Menghi, Vancouver, British Columbia

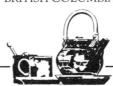

HOT CRAB AND CHEESE SANDWICH

Next to plain cracked crab trailed through lemon juice or mayonnaise, one of the best ways to serve crabmeat is as a hot sandwich, especially when it is combined with a cheese sauce.

2 Tbsp	butter	25 mL
2 Tbsp	flour	25 mL
1 tsp	dry mustard	5 mL
1 cup	milk	250 mL
1½ cups	grated old Cheddar cheese	375 mL
¼ tsp	cayenne	1 mL
6 oz	crabmeat, fresh or frozen, carefully cleaned of shell and cartilage fragments	175 g
1 Tbsp	mayonnaise	15 mL
4	thick slices whole wheat toast	4

1. Melt the butter in a saucepan. Add the flour and ½ tsp/2 mL dry mustard. Stir together to form a smooth paste and cook slowly for several minutes, but do not brown.

2. Stirring constantly, pour in the milk in a thin stream, cooking over medium heat until the sauce comes to a boil and thickens.

3. Add the cheese and cayenne, whisking until the cheese has melted. Remove from heat.

4. In a separate bowl, combine the crabmeat, mayonnaise and remaining dry mustard.

5. Spread the crab mixture on the toast, dividing it evenly.

6. Divide the 4 slices of toast between 2 ovenproof plates. Pour the cheese sauce over the toast and crabmeat. Place under a hot broiler for 1 minute, or until the top is lightly browned. Serve immediately.

Serves 2

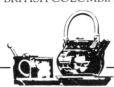

STIR-FRIED CRAB LEGS

Fresh crab legs and claws are infused with fresh garlic and ginger before being combined with sherry and soy sauce for a dish so messy and delicious that you may want to eat it in the bathtub. Or you can serve it with steamed rice and stir-fried vegetables. If you use frozen legs and claws, thaw them completely before cooking.

3 lb	crab legs and claws	1.5 kg
¼ cup	peanut oil	50 mL
2	cloves garlic, peeled	2
4	slices fresh ginger root	4
1 Tbsp	cornstarch	15 mL
½ cup	water	125 mL
2 Tbsp	soy sauce	25 mL
2 Tbsp	dry sherry	25 mL
1 tsp	granulated sugar	5 mL
1½ cups	sliced green onions	375 mL

1. Carefully crack the crab shells with a wooden mallet.

2. Heat a wok over high heat. Add the oil, garlic and ginger. Stir-fry for about 10 seconds, pressing the garlic and ginger to flavour the oil. Discard the garlic and ginger.

3. Add the cracked crab and stir for 10 minutes, or until the shells turn bright pink.

4. Combine the cornstarch, water, soy sauce, sherry and sugar. Add to the crab along with the green onions. Stir until the sauce is thick. Serve immediately.

Serves 2 to 4

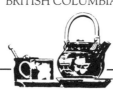

FRESH SALMON SCALLOPS WITH OYSTERS AND SORREL

This is salmon dressed up to go out at night. It is an ambitious recipe that assumes that you have gone out a few nights yourself and that you happen to have fish stock on hand (if you don't, use bottled clam juice). The oysters are soft and smooth and the sorrel is pleasantly sour-sharp. They are perfect playmates for west-coast salmon fillets. If you're going to do anything to fresh salmon besides poach it and serve it with hollandaise, this is a good bet. Buy the salmon from a good fish market where they can prepare it for this recipe.

1½ lb	fresh salmon, centre cut, skinned and boned	750 g
8	fresh oysters	8
6 cups	leaf spinach	1.5 L
¾ cup	fish stock	175 mL
⅔ cup	dry white wine	150 mL
⅔ cup	dry vermouth	150 mL
2	shallots, finely chopped	2
2 cups	sorrel leaves	500 mL
1 Tbsp	finely chopped parsley	15 mL
1 tsp	chopped fresh thyme leaves	5 mL
¼ cup	unsalted butter, cut into small pieces	50 mL
½ tsp	fresh lemon juice	2 mL
	Salt and freshly ground pepper to taste	
2 Tbsp	peanut oil	25 mL
	Crème Fraîche:	
1 cup	whipping cream	250 mL
2 Tbsp	cultured buttermilk	25 mL

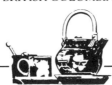

1. Prepare the crème fraîche by combining the whipping cream and buttermilk in a jar. Cover the jar, shake it, and let stand at room temperature overnight, or until thickened. Refrigerate until needed.

2. Cut the salmon lengthwise into 4 scallops. Flatten each slightly by pounding it gently with a meat cleaver between sheets of waxed paper.

3. Carefully open the oysters. Strain the juice into a bowl. Set the oysters aside, leaving them on the half shell.

4. Blanch the spinach by immersing it in boiling water for about 10 seconds, or until the leaves turn bright green. Immediately plunge the spinach in cold water. Dry.

5. Combine the fish stock, wine, vermouth and shallots in a heavy saucepan. Boil until reduced to about ¼ cup/50 mL.

6. Add the oyster juice and crème fraîche and simmer gently for 5 to 10 minutes, or until slightly thickened. Add the sorrel, parsley and thyme. Cook for 30 seconds.

7. Remove from heat and swirl in one-third of the butter. Add the lemon juice and season with salt and pepper.

8. Cook the blanched spinach in the remaining butter for 3 minutes.

9. Place the spinach on a serving platter and arrange the oysters in their shells around it. Put in a 275°F/140°C oven just to keep warm (no warmer or you'll cook the oysters).

10. Heat a large frying pan over high heat and lightly coat the bottom with peanut oil. Season the salmon with salt and pepper. Cook each piece in the hot oil for about 20 seconds per side (salmon should be undercooked).

11. Arrange the salmon on the spinach. Spoon some of the sauce over the oysters and salmon and serve the rest in a sauce boat.

Serves 4

—*William Tell Restaurant, Vancouver, British Columbia*

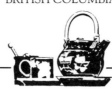

SALTSPRING LAMB WITH LEMON AND HERBS

The lemon-herb marinade in this recipe infuses the meat with a special pungency. Serve this with a steamed green vegetable and dry red wine.

1	leg of lamb, 5 to 6 lb/2.5 to 3 kg	1
1 Tbsp	unsalted butter	15 mL
4	carrots, scraped	4
4	stalks celery	4
2	large onions, quartered	2
1	large tomato, quartered	1
1 cup	water	250 mL
2 cups	beef stock	500 mL
	Marinade:	
¼ cup	olive oil	50 mL
¼ cup	fresh lemon juice	50 mL
2 Tbsp	grated lemon peel	25 mL
1	clove garlic, crushed	1
½ tsp	rosemary or 1 tsp/5 mL chopped fresh basil	2 mL
2	bay leaves	2
	Sauce:	
1 cup	dry red wine	250 mL
	Reserved marinade	
1 cup	whipping cream	250 mL
¼ cup	flour	50 mL

1. Combine all ingredients for the marinade. Pour over the lamb. Cover and refrigerate for 2 hours.

2. Remove the lamb from the marinade, then scrape the meat and dry it with paper towels. Reserve the marinade.

3. Add the butter to a large Dutch oven and brown the meat on all sides. Drain off the excess fat.

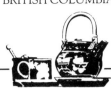

4. Add the carrots, celery, onions, tomato, water and stock. Simmer, covered, for 1½ hours over very low heat.

5. To prepare the sauce, blend together the wine, reserved marinade, whipping cream and flour. Pour over the lamb. Cover and simmer for 30 minutes.

6. Remove the meat to a platter. Strain the sauce and serve separately.

Serves 4

MOUNTAIN SQUAB WITH APPLES AND CIDER

Squabs are very young pigeons with meat that is denser and sweeter than chicken. They are tiny birds with little fat and must be prepared carefully so they won't dry out. Properly cooked, the mountain squab (now commercially raised on Vancouver Island) are a treat. They were included on the menu in 1984 when Canadian chefs competed in the International Culinary Olympics.

4	squab, dressed	4
⅓ cup	butter	75 mL
½ tsp	salt	2 mL
½ tsp	freshly ground pepper	2 mL
2	large apples, cut in half, cored but not peeled	2
1¼ cups	apple cider	300 mL

1. In a Dutch oven or large saucepan with a lid, brown the squab in the butter. Season with salt and pepper. Remove from the saucepan and set aside.

2. Slowly cook the apple halves in the pan drippings for 1 or 2 minutes, or until the cut surface is slightly brown. Remove the apples and set aside.

3. Return the squab to the saucepan. Add 1 cup/250 mL apple cider. Cover the pan and simmer the squab slowly in the cider for 1 hour.

4. Return the apples to the pan, spooning some of the pan juices over them. Continue cooking for 15 minutes.

5. Remove the squab and the apples from the pan and arrange them on a heated platter.

6. Deglaze the pan by adding ¼ cup/ 50 mL cider to the pan drippings. Swirl with a wire whisk, making sure you scrape up any brown bits clinging to the bottom. Taste for seasoning. Pour the sauce over the squab and apples.

Serves 2

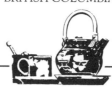

WHITE CHOCOLATE MOUSSE WITH RASPBERRY SAUCE

Among the chocolate desserts served in chocolate-mad Vancouver is this one, which is subtle in flavour and dramatic in colour contrast. Buy a good-quality white chocolate in a specialty store. If you wish, semisweet brown chocolate may be substituted.

3 oz	white chocolate	100 g
7 ½ tsp	warm milk	37 mL
1	egg white	1
½ tsp	fresh lemon juice	2 mL
pinch	salt	pinch
½ cup	whipping cream	125 mL
½ cup	chocolate shavings, brown or white	125 mL
	Fresh raspberries for garnish	
	Raspberry Sauce:	
1 cup	raspberries, fresh or frozen	250 mL
1 ½ tsp	water	7 mL
2 Tbsp	granulated sugar	25 mL
1 Tbsp	fresh lemon juice	15 mL
1 ½ tsp	light rum	7 mL

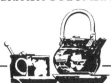

1. Melt the chocolate in the top of a double boiler. Add the warm milk, stirring until smooth. Cool the mixture to room temperature.

2. Beat the egg white with the lemon juice and salt until it forms stiff peaks. Beat the whipping cream until it forms soft peaks.

3. Fold the beaten egg white into the chocolate mixture. Then fold in the whipped cream, reserving a large spoonful for garnish.

4. Pour the mousse into 4 small soufflé dishes. Refrigerate, covered, overnight.

5. To prepare the raspberry sauce, combine the raspberries with the water in a saucepan. Bring to a boil and remove from heat.

6. In a food processor or blender, combine the raspberries with the sugar, lemon juice and rum and blend until smooth.

7. Strain sauce through a sieve.

8. To serve, unmould the mousse onto individual chilled plates. Garnish the top of each mousse with a ring of shaved chocolate. Surround with raspberry sauce. Top with a dab of whipped cream and a fresh raspberry.

Serves 4

—William Tell Restaurant,
Vancouver, British Columbia

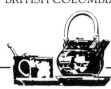

RUM PIE IN CHOCOLATE SHELL

This is a grown-up dessert, not too sweet and very sophisticated. Hold on to the recipe for the chocolate pie shell—it can be filled with ice cream, chocolate custard, chocolate mousse or fresh fruit and whipped cream. Use the best chocolate you can find for the shell.

There is no provision in this recipe for the egg whites you will have once you break the eggs to get the yolks, so you're on your own. I like to make meringues and fill them with pistachios to serve on the side.

	Chocolate Shell:	
2 Tbsp	shortening	25 mL
8 oz	semisweet chocolate	250 g
	Filling:	
6	egg yolks	6
scant 1 cup	granulated sugar	230 mL
1 Tbsp	unflavoured gelatine	15 mL
½ cup	cold water	125 mL
2 cups	whipping cream	500 mL
⅓ cup	dark rum	75 mL
2 Tbsp	chopped pistachio nuts	25 mL

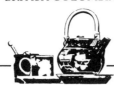

1. Preheat oven to 325°F/160°C.

2. To make the shell, line a 10-in/2-L glass pie plate with foil, smoothing the foil so there are no creases.

3. Add the shortening and chocolate chips. Melt them together in the oven for 10 minutes.

4. With a spatula, smear the melted chocolate and shortening over the bottom and sides of the foil until it forms a pie shell. If the chocolate is too runny, let it cool slightly.

5. Chill the chocolate shell in the refrigerator. When firmly chilled, carefully peel away the foil and rest the chocolate shell back in the pie plate or on a serving platter.

6. To make the filling, beat the egg yolks in a bowl until thick and light. Add the sugar and blend in.

7. Soften the gelatine in the cold water and dissolve slowly over low heat.

8. Beat the gelatine into the egg mixture. Place the bowl on a pan filled with cracked ice and stir until the mixture just begins to set.

9. Whip the cream until stiff. Fold into the egg mixture. Fold in the rum.

10. Pour the filling into the pie shell and sprinkle with pistachio nuts. Chill for about 2 hours, or until firm.

Serves 6

—Barbara Gordon, La Cachette,
Vancouver, British Columbia

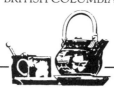

NANAIMO BARS

To call this confection just a layered chocolate cookie bar would be to deny its greater place in Canadian food mythology. No single dessert, with the possible exception of the Ontario butter tart, has enjoyed more speculation as to its origins. Theorists range from those who claim that it started with a recipe contest, to those who know for a fact that it was used to disguise illicit booze run from Canada to the United States during prohibition. And then there are heretics who claim that it doesn't come from Nanaimo at all!

	Bottom Layer:	
½ cup	butter	125 mL
¼ cup	granulated sugar	50 mL
⅓ cup	unsweetened cocoa	75 mL
1 tsp	vanilla	5 mL
1	egg, beaten	1
1 cup	unsweetened dessicated coconut	250 mL
2 cups	Graham wafer crumbs	500 mL
½ cup	chopped walnuts	125 mL
	Filling:	
¼ cup	butter	50 mL
2 Tbsp	milk	25 mL
2 Tbsp	vanilla custard or pudding powder (Bird's Custard Powder)	25 mL
2 cups	sifted icing sugar	500 mL
	Topping:	
4 oz	unsweetened chocolate	125 g
1 Tbsp	butter	15 mL

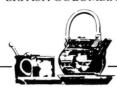

1. To make the bottom layer, melt the butter in a saucepan over low heat.

2. Add the sugar, cocoa, vanilla and egg. Cook, stirring over medium heat until the mixture thickens.

3. Remove from heat and stir in the coconut, crumbs and walnuts. Pat firmly into a buttered, 9-in/2-L square baking pan. Refrigerate for at least 1 hour.

4. To make the filling, cream the butter. Beat in the milk, custard powder and icing sugar. If the mixture is too thick to spread, add a few more drops of milk. Spread over the bottom layer and refrigerate for 30 minutes, or until firm.

5. For the top layer, melt the chocolate and butter in a dish set over hot water. Spread over the filling.

6. Before the chocolate hardens completely, cut into squares. Refrigerate for at least 1 hour.

Makes about 24 squares

—Nanaimo Chamber of Commerce,
Nanaimo, British Columbia

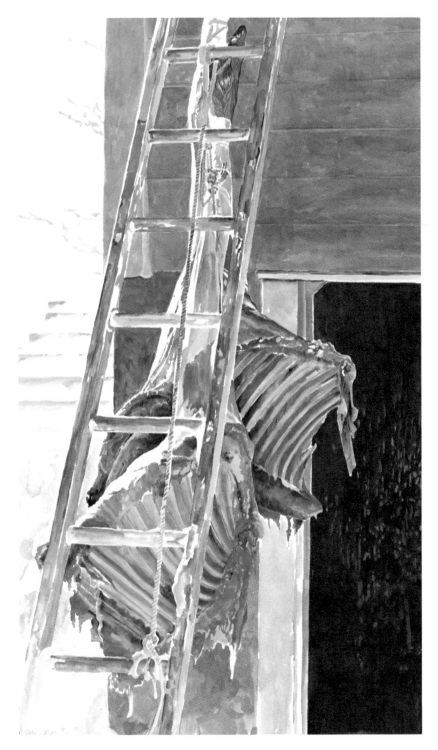

Moose—two forequarters

THE NORTH

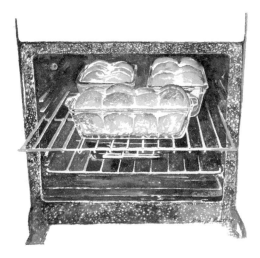

Northern Canada is not the place people think of for a gourmet holiday. Its culinary offerings seem limited to the clichés of Canadian food—pemmican, muktuk and moose stew.

I was intimidated by what I would find in the North. People who eat a lot of game rushed to assure me that I would love it once I tried it, and I always wondered why they felt they had to be so reassuring. Urbanites like myself who can barely sustain the idea of keeping a chicken in the backyard, or even preparing one that has not been clinically eviscerated, have a hard time understanding people who live somewhat closer to their food supply, sharing their gardens with their dinner.

To prepare for my first trip to the Yukon, I read books about cooking in the North. A government pamphlet called "Bear, Bacon and Boot Grease" gave step-by-step directions for "Seeking Out the Succulent Bear." Other writings comforted with instructions on how to gather the evening meal, but to my nervous ear they all sounded the same: "Grab a moose by the antlers and hit it between the eyes with an axe."

So apprehensive was I about eating the food of the North that I took a box of chocolates on the four-hour flight from Vancouver to Whitehorse. The night I arrived, I made a note in my eating diary to find bannock and bear. The next day I found both. But I also found croissants and cappuccino.

There were further surprises. I was promised the best cinnamon buns I could sink my teeth into in a motel near Dawson City. The best pizza was in Rankin Inlet and, if I should feel the urge, I could have quiche in Yellowknife.

And who knows what else I'd find if I took the years it would take to cover the area. Northern Canada is enormous. The Northwest Territories alone cover more than 1.3 million square miles, an area so huge that it is divided into three districts, each big enough to call a continent. The Territories lie like a roof top over five Canadian provinces, but they are sparsely populated by three major groups: Indian, Inuit and "other." One-quarter of the population of about 40,000 lives in Yellowknife.

By comparison, the Yukon is a small town, yet it is more than twice the size of the British Isles. It has a mere 500,000 square miles, plus a few. Its total population is about 25,000, most of it concentrated around White-horse and Dawson City.

Even for Canadians who have come to accept as commonplace vast distances between major centres, the North is overwhelming. It takes as long to fly from Whitehorse in the Yukon to Yellowknife in the Northwest Territories as it does to fly from Toronto to Los Angeles. And it costs more. The sparseness between is wonderful when you're sightseeing and intimi-dating if you're hungry. If you try to rent a car in Whitehorse to drive the glorious route to Inuvik, you will be told to expect long stretches of uninterrupted wilderness and be asked for an $800 drop-off charge.

In a sense, northern Canada has as many regions as all of the rest of Canada. Foods eaten in one part of the North may be unknown in another, and even for foods that are common throughout, there are areas of specialty. Around Inuvik there are more caribou and Arctic char than there are around Whitehorse, where they get more salmon and moose. In Old Crow in the Yukon, most of the foods, particularly small game, are prepared very simply by being boiled in plain water. But near Baffin Island they like their delicacies less delicate. There, I'm told, a popular treat is prepared by leaving a small bird to rot behind a rock until it begins to smell and tastes like Roquefort cheese. Another delicacy is partially digested shrimp gathered from the stomach of a freshly killed fish. It tastes, apparently, just like pâté, though I have taken this information on faith alone.

But in the larger, easily serviced communities where planes land and trucks drive, eating habits have much in common with those in large communities to the south. Although their isolation may cause residents to suffer less the vicissitudes of culinary fashion than in other parts of Canada, they are still influenced by food trends that have affected the menus of all Canadians. Though many foods, particularly packaged and canned foods, may be standard, prices aren't. Because of the distance, food prices in the North are much higher. The official Canadian food basket may cost at least twice as much in Yellowknife as it does in Edmonton.

Generally, all of Canada is affected in eating habits more by neighbours to the south than to the east or west. On a smaller scale, the same is true in the North. Because the Yukon is relatively close to British Columbia, some of the foods and the way they are treated are similar. Salmon bakes, sourdough bread and Alaska king crab are found wherever tourists roam, from San Francisco to British Columbia, Alaska and the Yukon. In Yellowknife, there are perogies and the other Ukrainian specialties that reflect its proximity to Alberta.

Throughout the north, there's a lot of socializing over food. "There's a fair emphasis on oral gratification among people in what might be considered pretty barren country," one former resident of Yellowknife told me. There's also a lot of socializing over drink. The Yukon boasts the highest alcohol consumption per capita in Canada. The price of booze is high, and although costs have been equalized throughout the North to compensate for the demands of distribution to far-flung regions, many residents keep their own costs down by preparing home brew. Very common in the Northwest Territories is hootch made with raisins and yeast, which can be found brewing in bathtubs. Homemade wine is also popular. One well-travelled Canadian who spent several years in Yellowknife told me that the finest wine he ever drank was made from cranberries picked just outside of town.

In Whitehorse one resident estimated that in his town alone there were thirteen taverns, "not including those attached to hotels." They are open seven days a week. The bars are the social centres of town. There, games, stories and, very frequently, punches are traded.

The hale-fellow heartiness of the bars contributes to the image of the rough-and-tumble North, where people tend to take matters into their own hands—in bars, and elsewhere. Take the Taku Grill in Whitehorse, for example.

The Taku is in a hotel in the centre of town—a hotel much like other hotels in the North that have rooms, a saloon and a somewhat shabby restaurant with booths and counter stools. When Claude Aube went into the Taku one morning at 6 a.m., he was prepared to ignore the surroundings and even the fact that the food he had been served there the day before had been cold. But on this particular morning, injury was added to insult. The hash browns were like ice. And this time he wasn't going to take it. He complained to the cook.

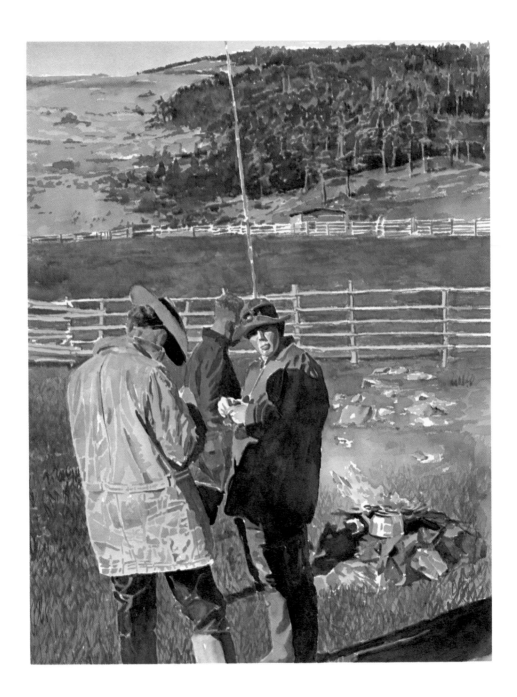

Boys going fishing "across the bay"

*Early morning fishing trips in late spring. Boys with
flies stuck in their hat brims, long rubber boots, tea
boiling over a little fire, the smell of wet alder
bushes—dreams of trout. (M.P.)*

The cook had his own troubles. Weary of complaints, James Collins responded to Aube's demands by emptying a bottle of Tabasco sauce on the potatoes. "Hot enough for ya now?" he asked.

Aube, in fact, was himself very hot. He followed the cook to the kitchen. Collins saw him coming and grabbed a carving knife. Bursting through the kitchen doors, he stabbed Aube in the heart.

Aube died and Collins got life imprisonment. In the North, breakfast is a serious business.

Unlike the many meals in the North that I approached with some trepidation, I heartily looked forward to breakfast. The northern breakfast is famous for its excess. At many hotels, the breakfast special is served on an oval platter that would hold a large roast chicken and veggies. Lining and overlapping the platter are enormous flapjacks, puffy and dense with milk, eggs and flour. On them lie eggs, done to order, and on top of that is a mound of bacon or sausages. All crevices and spare corners on this Vesuvius of food are taken up with plastic tubs of pancake syrup. Coffee is strong, limitless and very necessary for anyone facing such a mammoth meal at an early hour.

Such breakfasts had their beginnings in times when people ate them early and then headed to the hills to shoot bears. Most of the time they were unsure of where their next meal was coming from or how much strenuous work might be required for them to get it. Northern breakfasts are not designed for tourists who rise late and slow, then spend the rest of the day on buses viewing the frontier from behind glass shields.

In the North, game is the basic foodstuff, so unless you eat three breakfasts a day, it's hard to avoid it. City folks have a thing about game. Invite me for dinner and tell me we're having roast bear and I get a picture of candles in the dining room and, in the kitchen, a whole hairy bear lying in a roasting pan, its paws in the air. We urbanites have disguised our blood lust with euphemisms. We don't roast a cow. We have a steak or roast beef. We don't have a baby calf newly weaned from its mom. We have veal. When they do change the name of meat in the North, it's because they hope to sell it to people who don't like to eat animals they've seen on Walt Disney. Muskox, a meat popular in the Northwest Territories, is called polar beef by the people who sell it to tourist hotels.

In the North, game is simply called wild meat. It is not a curiosity dish but an important part of the daily menu, sometimes served at every meal. Elsie Netro, an Athabascan Loucou Indian from Old Crow, described to me a typical daily menu when she was growing up. Breakfast would be porridge or eggs and fried meat; lunch would be boiled or fried meat and bannock; dinner would be meat and berries.

Call it game or call it wild meat, call it muskox or polar beef—it doesn't matter. Because when you call it, it doesn't come. You have to go and catch it. Perhaps hunting a wild animal is no less fraught with danger than Saturday morning at the supermarket, but somehow it sounds tougher to me.

Like shoppers and gatherers of food everywhere, hunters have consumer hints. As Don Sawatsky who lives near Whitehorse explained over coffee in a nice restaurant one morning, "You gotta get them right. I once saw a nice bull moose. Dropped him with one shot right here," he said, pointing to a spot behind his ear. "It was the easiest shot and the toughest thing I ever ate. You have to stalk them carefully. Some people feel if they're startled the meat gets tough. The Indians, mind you, like the taste of a startled animal, but I think it's too wild. Anyway, once you get the moose, you take the hide off and douse the meat with pepper, then hang it for a week or so. It's always a judgement call about when to shoot and how long to hang it, but you do get a feel for it after a while."

And, just like my sister and I always used to fight over the turkey neck, there are favourite parts of the moose. The nose in particular, which is roasted—and served whole.

In the Yukon, the main meat has always been moose, a dense and very lean beef-like animal. Elsie Netro's husband bags one in the fall and parcels it carefully so that it lasts through the winter. The Netros vary their meat diet with grouse and rabbit and occasionally with chicken and pork they may pick up at a store on the way home from their jobs as teacher and engineer. And although it is illegal to sell game, if you go to the right bars and talk to the right people, Don Sawatsky says you can find it: "You go to a bar in the fall when the hunt's at its peak. Drop it around that you'd like some meat and maybe a day or so later, someone will knock at your door."

However squeamish you may feel about eating wild meat for the first time, once you've had it, you'll probably miss it. Caribou, the meat most popular in the Northwest Territories, has won that kind of loyalty. One Toronto man who lived in Yellowknife for years, longingly described Caribou Stroganoff, a dish that apparently became popular when the Russians owned the Arctic. It's essentially the same as Beef Stroganoff, but made with caribou meat, it has its own special flavour.

Because caribou is so lean and mild, it can be easily substituted for beef or veal. To initiate me to the meat, my friend Gail made cabbage rolls with ground caribou, then later brazenly served a caribou roast with couscous as a side dish at a dinner party. It was a large roast, which she cooked pink at the bone and flavoured only with salt, pepper and huge chunks of garlic stuck randomly into the meat. Over the top she laid strips of bacon that yielded the fat to moisturize the flesh during cooking. It was very nice.

Fat is nearly always required when cooking wild meat because the meat is so lean from all that running around in the bush. Caribou is a beautiful meat. Raw, its colour is a burnished burgundy-brown. There is no visible fat. It has the texture of lean sirloin, but when you hold it up, it flaps like a piece of liver. It should be cooked rare and tender. Nelson Lewis, a professionally trained chef whose specialty is northern game, prefers caribou curried with apples, oranges, bananas, raisins and coconut and served in a sauce spiked with beer and apple cider. People who have eaten caribou head (the tongue and the brain are apparently the best parts) tell me that it is also a real treat.

Lewis likes moose heart, too—stuffed and cooked with beer. But about bear meat, he is rhapsodic. Like many wild game cooks, Lewis is very fond of bear fat, which is so loved that it is kind of an elixir in the North. Rendered, it makes the best French fries and the best pie crusts in the world. It has uses outside the kitchen, too, as a hair conditioner and leather softener. In spite of the fact that the meat has such a strong taste, bear fat, properly rendered with water, has no particular flavour.

Bears in the bush are reluctant to give up their fat—or any other part of their bodies. Lewis, who teaches people how to cook in the bush, instills in his students respect for their subject with some quick facts. Black bears are so strong, according to Lewis, that they can run up and down trees like squirrels, can push boulders around like peanuts and can run about thirty-five miles per hour.

Nelson Lewis's courses are offered mostly for people who provide food for bush workers. This is an especially daunting task because meals are so important when workers are isolated in the bush with no other diversion. The people who prepare food for the bush workers must be particularly well trained and resourceful because they cannot rely on materials that have to be carried in and out. They rely on many cooking and gathering methods taught to them by the Indians.

Whatever the trials of bush cooks, they are spared the cruelty of metric. Their measurements are more basic. A "handful" is the quantity obtained by filling the hand as full as possible. "Two fingers" is a measurement used for dry materials like flour or baking powder. Hold the number of fingers required close together and scoop out the material. But if the instructions call for "one finger of fat," then use the little finger as a scoop, taking as much fat as will stay in the bend of the finger.

Bush cooks must also know things of no concern to any other cook in the world, such as how to keep bears away from the kitchen. Lewis teaches that there must be no cooking smell or any remnants of dinner. Camp cooks must also know how to shoot—not just to get game, but to protect themselves and the camp, since they are there by themselves during the day.

After my first taste of black bear, I felt I had to protect myself against the animal alive or cooked. Sour cream bear was one of the recipes Nelson Lewis prepared for me the evening I went to his place for dinner. I thought that it tasted like old sheep and I loathed it. But I loved the muskox chops, thick and juicy at the bone, which fell apart at the touch of my fork, and the cold poached salmon that had been pulled from the Taku River and garnished with fireweed, a local wild plant. The moose pot pie was completely wonderful, the moose meat subtle, almost sweet, with the texture of beef chuck. No wonder I loved it.

Sometimes when people are trying to convince you how much you'd like some funny meat, they'll tell you that it tastes just like something else that doesn't scare you. When they are trying to coax you to eat wild meat, they'll compare it to the most domesticated meat that comes to mind, usually chicken. But when well-meaning people promised me that squirrel and porcupine tasted like chicken, I said, thanks, but I'll have chicken.

I couldn't avoid them if I lived in the North, where small game is an important supplement to the daily diet. When I asked Elsie Netro how one would go about catching and cooking a porcupine, she assured me there was nothing to it. "First of all you club them instead of shooting them because you don't want pellets in the meat. You have to move fast to club them because they're quick. Then you singe off the quills and keep scraping until they're all off. The singeing adds flavour to the meat, just like when you brown chicken. Wash the porcupine, then cut it up into parts—thighs, head, breasts and forearms. Then you boil it until it's done."

There are many northern specialties that are surely an acquired taste. Muktuk, the inside skin membrane between the fat and the meat of a whale, is eaten like popcorn by Inuit in the Northwest Territories and is probably no more horrific to them than the chicken livers all squished up with butter and brandy that I like on toast. But I found the stuff very fishy, with a texture like erasers.

Considering the caloric advantages to eating game, I'm surprised it didn't catch on ages ago. For example, 3½ oz. of polar bear has 130 calories, while 4 oz. of beef hamburger has 364. And 3½ oz. of caribou has 120 calories, while a 3-oz. lamb chop has 230. You may wish to stay away from beaver, which has 408 calories in a 3½-oz. serving, though you may

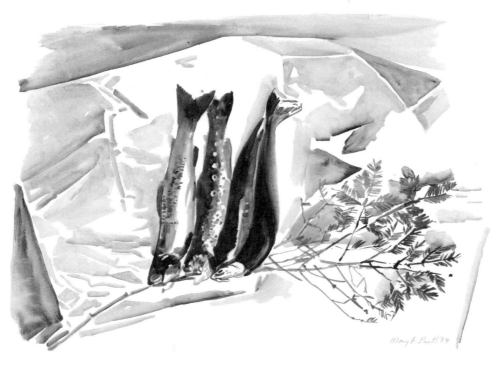

Four trout on a spruce "gad"

From the river that flows by our front garden, my children brought me many trout strung on spruce "gads." The only reason catches remained fairly small was the rule that each child had to clean what he caught. (M.P.)

be interested in the popular beaver tail soup, which is much like consomme. Roast a cleaned and skinned beaver tail in a hot oven or bake in foil in a fire for 30 minutes. Cut it up and put in a soup pot. Cover the meat with water and bring to a simmer. Add onions, carrots, celery, wild onions and a bay leaf. Simmer until the water is reduced by half. Season with salt and pepper and eat it hot or cold. (When it's cold, it gels like consomme.)

Game is now more widely available than it used to be, and there are many farms where it is raised and harvested. The meat may not have the true flavour of the wild, but domestication does mean that restaurants all over Canada can include game on their fall menus. At Fenton's in Toronto, where it would be difficult to imagine the nattily dressed proprietors out stalking deer, partridge and venison pies are served in November. Both meats are from farms. ULU Foods in Inuvik distributes nearly every available kind of fish and game, including Arctic char, northern pike, caribou and muskox, though most of their customers are hotels and restaurants in the North. Otherwise selling game is illegal, and you can only get it if you hunt or receive it as a gift.

I found other foods that are gathered in the wild to be much more palatable. Elsie spoke of cranberries, which come either from high bush or low bush plants. High bush cranberries are sweet, like red currants, while the low bush berries are harder and stronger, like those we get in supermarkets. She spoke with rapture of salmonberries, sometimes called knuckleberries, which she says are like huge orange raspberries, but taste even better. The cranberries are often made into pies, but the knuckleberries seldom get past the picking.

There are vegetables, too. Wild onions are like leeks, and are especially good fried in great amounts and served with meat. Willow tips taste like crunchy breakfast cereal; spruce tips can be steeped in water for a drink; woolly lousewort can be used in a salad or boiled as greens, since its roots taste like young carrots.

Sometimes the wild onions and berries would be served at Elsie's as part of a huge family dinner. Such dinners have a hierarchy of table service that would do much to prevent middle-age spread: elders are served first, then children and finally parents. The family doesn't necessarily all eat at the table. They take a plate from a central table and find a spot somewhere in the house.

Elsie's favourite family feast includes caribou ribs and Alaska king crab legs—a northern version of surf n' turf.

There are those in the North who feel that the Americans got the best of the gastronomic deals in Alaska, where the caribou is sweeter because of the grass it grazes on and where succulent huge crab legs are there for the asking. But we make up for it with the fabulous fish of the Canadian North. That is one kind of game we can all swallow.

The fish of the North is superb. Chilly waters seem to make the flesh richer and its flavour more intense. In the Yukon and Northwest Territories there is inconnu, so-called because no one knows what its real name is, though the Russians have referred to it as white salmon or Nelma. It is caught in northern rivers only in the late fall, when sometimes it must be fished through the ice. The inconnu is a large fish (a small one is eight to ten pounds), firm fleshed and very rich with a taste that has been compared to cool fresh cream.

And people who have spent time fishing where it is chilly talk ecstatically about loche liver, which refers to the northern delicacy made from the liver and sometimes the roe of the freshwater cod that is caught in the small streams of the Mackenzie Delta in October. Sometimes the liver is mixed with ground ptarmigan gizzard, the roe and liver are pan-fried in lard or butter and served hot for a special treat.

I had heard rapturish stories of fresh fish hoisted right out of chilly northern waters and pan-fried soon after the hook has been pulled from the gill. So it was with much anticipation that I once joined several experienced fishermen to troll for northern pike. We spent several hours trailing lines through calm waters one beautiful August morning and netted a couple of dozen fish for a reward. We carried these fish to the shore of an uninhabited island for the "shore lunch" we had been anticipating all morning. As the men filleted the fish and I chopped vegetables, I anticipated the fish being cooked with butter and maybe some garlic, but so very lightly that nothing would mask the sweet taste of fish just out of the water.

Well, I still haven't tasted fish cooked that way. The cook took each of the fillets and placed it in a bag filled with Shake 'n Bake, shook it and, to my horror, added it to a pan bubbling with melted margarine.

Nevertheless, the fish was wonderful, falling into soft flakes at the touch of the lake-rinsed forks, crunchy at the edges from its fast frying. Later, sitting at the edge of the rock, feet dangling in the lake with the water lapping at our bare feet, sun keeping our food and us hot, our guide said, "You know, it's at times like these I feel sorry for the Queen. She can never eat like this."

Indeed she can't.

Frances Macalquham, a noted expert on fish and game cookery, claimed that properly catching, storing and cleaning the fish is as important, if not more important, than cooking it, since no recipe in the world can overcome bad field work. She offered a few tips. Kill the fish as soon as it's caught, not only because it's humane, but because flesh deteriorates more rapidly in fish left to die slowly. Don't put fish in pails of water or let them drag along behind the boat, because water impedes the natural drainage of the fish. Besides, the relatively warmer water at the surface interferes with rigor mortis. The fish should be bled immediately; either cut its throat or simply cut off its head. (Don't throw away the heads, they make good stocks and chowders.)

Keep the fish cool, and cook and eat it quickly. Should someone hand you what they promise is their fresh catch, check it carefully. The flesh should spring back to finger pressure; the scales should be firmly attached and glisten like sequins; the eyes should be well-rounded and protruding, not sunken; no bones should stick through the flesh on the inside cavity of a gutted fish; the gills should be bright red. Take a sniff at the gills. The fish should smell mild, light and fresh. A saltwater fish will have a slight trace of iodine.

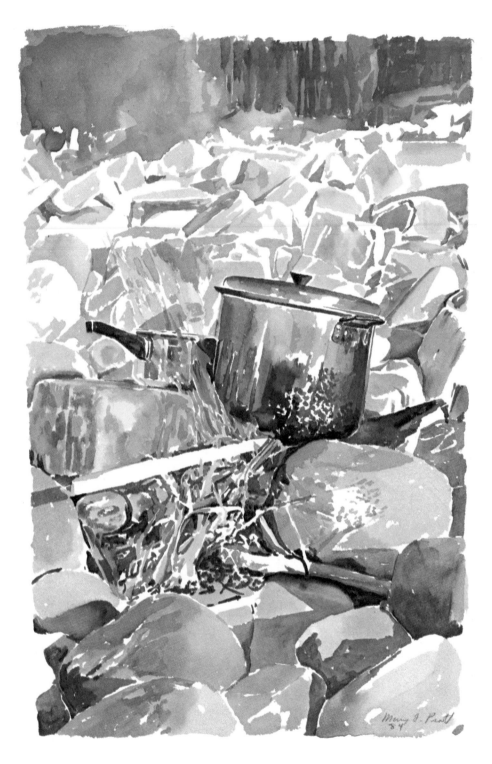

Lobsters are in this pot

Northern Canada has always had a kind of romantic appeal for fishermen and seekers of peace and untrammeled nature. To be there in the summertime is to find it all. During the month of July, the light leaves for barely an hour at around three in the morning. One might think that residents get used to having constant daylight, and go to sleep at eleven and eat their meals at the same hours as they do during the rest of the year. But the light affects them in odd ways. In July people pack picnic lunches and head up into the mountains for a light dinner and a swim at a warm-water spring at midnight. In town, they might go to a restaurant for a meal of reindeer meat or Alaska king crab legs and a bottle of wine, leaving the restaurant into bright sunshine at 11 p.m. It feels as if the day is just beginning. In fact, sleeping is very difficult. When the sun is shining outside at two in the morning, you feel like a child who has been put to bed early. It turns the calmest people into insomniacs.

But that's the summer. For the greater part of the year, it's dark and very cold. People want soups and foods that are fatter to keep them warm. Lean fish are fed to the dogs, while fatter fish, like trout, are saved for their masters. There is much reliance in all communities on canned vegetables and fruits in the winter. Powdered foods are used, too, especially powdered eggs and milk.

Of course, it's easier to preserve some things in nature's freezer. Fresh foods last longer in the North. In *The Northern Cookbook*, author Eleanor Ellis advises that frozen oranges, grapefruit or lemons may be coated with ice to prevent them from drying out. She also advises that if you add a spoonful of salt to your last rinse water, your laundry won't freeze to your clothesline. Or, "When melting snow, you need a layer of water in the bottom of the pot to prevent the pot from burning."

None of these frosty realities seem to deter pioneers looking for a new life in Canada's North, though today's immigrants are as likely to be well-educated urbanites seeking an alternative to the rat race as grizzled gold-panners seeking fast fortune. These pioneers bring with them sophisticated ways of eating and cooking, and quickly incorporate them into their new lives. That is why throughout northern Canada there are restaurants that seem at odds with the environment—establishments more likely on a street corner in downtown Toronto than on a dirt road in Inuvik.

One of Canada's best bakeries is the Alpine Bakery in Whitehorse, operated by Suat Tuzlak who came to the Yukon several years ago to cross-country ski and decided he liked it better there than in Calgary where he was living and Yugoslavia where he had lived before that. Suat had trained as a mechanical engineer. Now he engineers pastries and breads, no mean

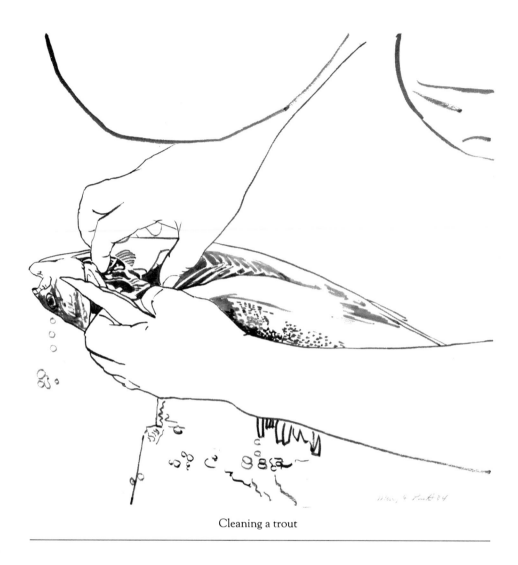

Cleaning a trout

task in the North where temperatures and altitudes routinely threaten the volatile live yeast he uses in his baking.

Tuzlak makes bannock, to be sure, but he makes it like a French patissière—light with flaky layers and laced with Cheddar, so that it flakes in your mouth and tastes like shortbread. But he also makes sourdough bread, so indigenous to the North that people who have lived there all their lives are called "sourdoughs." (People who have not yet spent a winter are called "cheesecakes," which has a slightly different connotation in the North than it has in the South.)

Next door to the Alpine Bakery is The No Pop Sandwich Shop, Whitehorse's only bistro. Here Arthur Giovannizzo, an ex-social worker from Vancouver, serves he-man sandwiches, cappuccino and fresh straw-

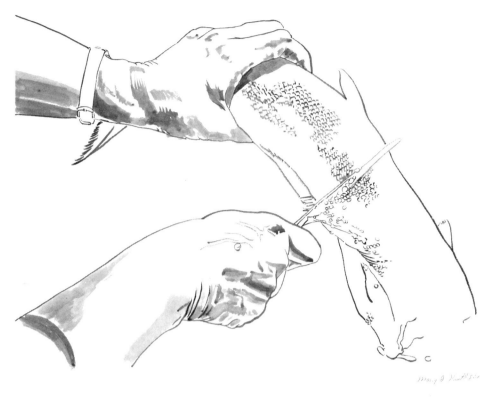

Scaling a trout

berry ice cream made down the street by a couple of kids who like earning extra pocket money. "When I moved here I figured, if there can be cappuccino in Kitsilano and Rosedale, why not in Whitehorse? It was a struggle at first, but now," he says, "it's a breeze."

So much a breeze that he is considering opening similar cappuccino-espresso bars in small towns all over western Canada. In towns like Whitehorse, he says, people gravitate to the kitchen at a party. So he finds that his homey place is where the town's three dozen lawyers talk over land claims, and local shop owners discuss the price of lettuce.

Giovannizzo defines himself as a reconstructed hippie, one of many free spirits seeking escape from urban demands and pollution. Those who live on the land, trying to grow what they can and eating pure foods are called "bush bunnies." The game that is so basic to the diet of indigenous northerners is anathema to them.

Living life as a vegetarian in the North is no small challenge in a land where the growing season is short and topsoil is scarce. Nevertheless, there are two health food stores in Whitehorse and, when I last checked, an

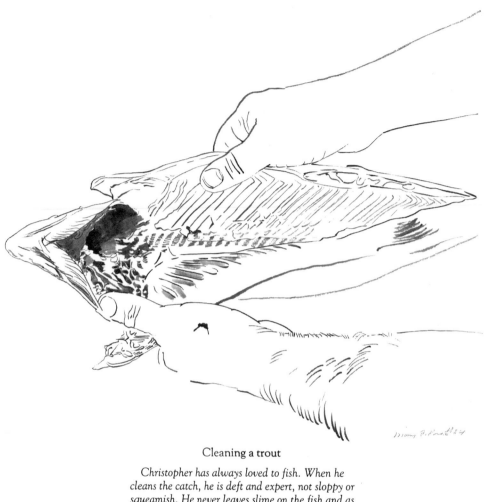

Cleaning a trout

*Christopher has always loved to fish. When he
cleans the catch, he is deft and expert, not sloppy or
squeamish. He never leaves slime on the fish and as
a result they are delicious. (M.P.)*

attempt to form the Whitehorse Vegetarian Society was meeting with
success. Members get together for potluck suppers once a month.

The gastronomic guru for the Yukon's reformed eating movement is Dr.
Philip Brannigan, the town's mayor and a medical doctor. He had long
preached the benefits of holistic medicine and alternative lifestyles which
the bemused medical establishment of Whitehorse tolerated until he
began to practice psychic surgery—a method of routing out sickness by
thinking rather than cutting.

Despite his loss of hospital privileges and the disdain in which the
medical community holds him, he claims to be the leading local doctor,
with one-quarter of the population as his patients. Many of the area's bush
bunnies speak of him with reverence.

Brannigan finds trying to reform people's eating habits no small task ("People will change their partners, their jobs and even their country before they'll change their diets"). But he claims some success. "When I first came here from Alberta, this was an affluent, hard-drinking and meat-eating community, but people have shifted now. They're more aware of nutrition, and even though it's expensive they do have vegetables."

They also have granola and tofu and carob. And Yin and Yang. Dr. Brannigan matches his patients to the kinds of foods they eat using the Chinese theory of Yin and Yang. Yang, he told me, are aggressive foods that have high colour, like red meat and cayenne. Yin are pacifying foods and include rice, vegetables and fruit.

Much of his challenge has existed because the North is inclined to be Yang, though there are regional differences: "The Northwest Territories are much more Yang than the Yukon," he told me, "and the farther north you go in the Northwest Territories, the more Yang it gets."

I spent an evening with some of Dr. Brannigan's followers at their spiritual headquarters in the mountains near Whitehorse. On one daylit night we sipped herbal tea and ate rice crackers with no additives. I found it quite a relief from muktuk. And easier to prepare than porcupine.

Rice crackers, cappuccino and quiche admittedly have made surviving in the rough much easier for us cheesecakes. But I hope my favourites will always be there as well: the breakfasts, berries and bannock. And the fish and caribou.

But the next time someone invites me to hunt and then eat black bear, I'm going to look for a nice restaurant that takes Diner's Club.

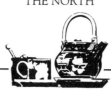

CHECKERBOARD CHOWDER

This hearty chowder takes its name from the variety of fish that go into it. It is often made by fishermen who have odd bits and pieces of fish left in the freezer at the end of a season.

2	medium onions, chopped	2
1	green or red pepper, chopped	1
4	cloves garlic, chopped	4
2	stalks celery, chopped	2
¼ cup	vegetable oil	50 mL
¼ cup	olive oil	50 mL
4 lb	fish fillets, any kind	2 kg
6	tomatoes, peeled, seeded and chopped, or 1 28-oz/796-mL tin	6
1	bay leaf	1
6 cups	hot water	1.5 L
2 cups	white wine	500 mL
1 Tbsp	lemon juice	15 mL
¼ cup	finely chopped parsley	50 mL
1 tsp	fennel seed	5 mL
1 tsp	salt	5 mL
½ tsp	freshly ground pepper	2 mL
24	clams or mussels	24

1. In a large soup pot, cook the onions, green pepper, garlic and celery in the vegetable and olive oils.

2. Add the fish, tomatoes, bay leaf and hot water. Bring to a boil, reduce the heat and simmer slowly for 20 minutes.

3. Add the remaining ingredients, except for the clams or mussels. Continue to simmer for a further 15 minutes.

4. Add the clams or mussels. Simmer until the shells open. Adjust seasonings.

Serves 6 to 8

MUD-BAKED PICKEREL WITH WILD RICE STUFFING

This Indian method of cooking fish or game in the bush ensures that the meat will be tender and succulent. One of the advantages is that the skin and scales of the fish stick to the mud after the fish is cooked, leaving a feast of clean meat. The best clay for this kind of cookery will be damp and dense enough that when you squeeze a handful, it will stick together without cracking.

The fish for this recipe must be drawn, but the head should be left on. A clay baker in the right shape for the fish may be substituted for the clay.

If you are going whole hog, use bear fat instead of bacon, wild onions and toss some bulrush roots into the stuffing.

1	whole pickerel or other whitefish, 2 to 3 lb/1 to 1.5 kg	1
2 tsp	salt	10 mL
1	small onion, diced	1
1 Tbsp	bacon fat	15 mL
1 cup	cooked wild rice	250 mL
1/2 tsp	pepper	2 mL
1 tsp	chopped fresh dill or other herb	5 mL

1. Clean the fish, leaving the skin and head on. Wash in cold water. Wipe clean and rub the salt into the cavity.

2. Cook the onion in the bacon fat. Add the wild rice, pepper and fresh dill.

3. Stuff the fish with the wild rice stuffing. Tie it together with a piece of cotton string or pliable root.

4. Roll out 2 pieces of clay about 3/4 in/2 cm thick and large enough to hold the fish. Place the fish in the centre of one of the clay cakes. Place the other cake on top and seal around the edges.

5. Rake out some coal from the fire, cover the mud pack with coals and put more wood on the fire. Cook for at least 1 hour.

6. Remove the mud pack from the coals, crack open. Eat directly from the mud shell.

Serves 2 to 3

—From Wilderness Cooking *by Berndt Berglund and Clare Bolsby (Toronto: Pagurian Press, 1973)*

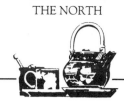

ARCTIC CHAR WITH HERBED MAYONNAISE

Fished from the icy streams of the Canadian Arctic and sub-Arctic, the Arctic char has no scales. It is silvery pink with beautiful large spots of pink on its belly and sides. It can weigh up to 20 lb/10 kg though the smaller fish are best for eating. It is a fish that tends to dry very easily, so care must be taken not to overcook it.

Arctic char is often best simply poached and served with mayonnaise sauces flavoured with herbs. Because of its beauty, it is dramatic served cold and whole, as it is in this recipe. For buffets, whole poached char is sometimes garnished with tiny penguins made from hard-boiled eggs.

1	whole Arctic char, 10 to 12 lb/5 to 6 kg, thawed	1
2 qt	milk	2 L
1 Tbsp	chopped fresh tarragon	15 mL
	Herbed Mayonnaise:	
1 cup	mayonnaise	250 mL
1 tsp	chopped fresh dill	5 mL
1 tsp	chopped fresh basil	5 mL
1/2 tsp	chopped fresh tarragon	2 mL
	Penguins:	
4	hard-boiled eggs, peeled	4
6	black olives	6
4	white almonds, in pieces, for eyes and mouths	4
1	large carrot, sliced in thin coins	1

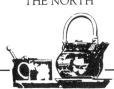

1. Wrap the entire char in cheesecloth and lay it in a poacher large enough to hold it so that it doesn't bend.

2. Combine the milk and the tarragon. Pour around the fish. The milk should come halfway up the sides of the fish.

3. Bring to a boil, then reduce the heat to a bare simmer. Poach the fish very gently, allowing 5 to 8 minutes per lb/500 g. Be careful not to overcook.

4. Remove the char from the milk bath still wrapped in the cheesecloth (the cheesecloth will keep the fish intact and prevent milk scum from settling).

5. Allow the char to cool and then remove the cheesecloth. Lay the char on a serving platter (you can remove the skin if you prefer, but it can be quite pretty if it is still intact).

6. To make the herbed mayonnaise, combine the mayonnaise with the fresh dill, basil and tarragon.

7. Serve the fish with the herbed mayonnaise. Garnish the platter with penguins.

8. Dress the eggs as penguins, using toothpicks to attach the olive and carrot pieces. The black olives become the heads and wings; the almond pieces become the eyes and mouths; the carrot coins become feet.

Serves 8 to 10

PTARMIGAN WITH FRESH CRANBERRIES AND WHITE WINE

When a recipe requires that the bird, fish or game be "dressed," what it really means is that the meat is "undressed"—its guts and feathers, hide or scales have been removed and the meat readied for cooking.

Like most game birds, ptarmigan has lean and dense flesh, which requires the addition of fat and gentle steam from braising. Here the bacon lends not only the fat, but a salty smokiness. The freshly popped berries and the white wine add sweet-tartness. Domestic squab or Cornish game hens can easily be substituted for the ptarmigan. This recipe is accomplished on a stove top or campfire; no oven is required.

4	slices side bacon	4
8	ptarmigan or squab or 4 Cornish game hens, dressed	8
1	medium onion, diced	1
2	cloves garlic, minced	2
1	stalk celery, with leaves, sliced on diagonal	1
2	carrots, sliced on diagonal	2
1 tsp	salt	5 mL
1 tsp	freshly ground pepper	5 mL
1 cup	dry white wine	250 mL
1 cup	fresh cranberries	250 mL
1 Tbsp	brown sugar	15 mL
1 Tbsp	fresh lemon juice	15 mL

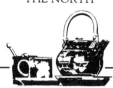

1. In a Dutch oven or large heavy saucepan with a lid, cook the bacon until medium-crisp. Drain bacon on paper towels.

2. Brown the birds in the rendered bacon fat, flattening them in the pan as they brown.

3. Add the onion, garlic, celery and carrots and continue to cook until the onion becomes translucent. Add the salt and pepper and stir them in.

4. Add the white wine, scraping the pot to include the delicious browned bits clinging to the bottom. Cover the pot and simmer the birds over low to medium heat until they are tender. This will take 1 to 1½ hours, depending on the heat.

5. Add the fresh cranberries. Replace the lid and simmer for about 10 minutes, or until the berries pop.

6. Stir the brown sugar and lemon juice into the pot, coating the birds.

7. Serve immediately on a platter of wild or brown rice. Garnish the birds with the slices of reserved bacon.

Serves 4 to 6

—*Nelson Lewis, Whitehorse, Yukon*

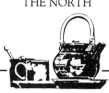

MUSKOX MEAT LOAF WITH QUAIL EGGS

Muskox has been considered an endangered species, but may now be purchased quite legally from sources in the Northwest Territories who have farmed it in accordance with the law and sometimes sell it under the name of Polar Beef. It has a lean, beefy flavour. A muskox chop is about the size of a large veal chop, but its meat is darker.

Ground game is used in the North much the same way ground beef is used—in spaghetti sauces, for hamburgers or just pan fried in a hash with whatever vegetable is available. Here it becomes meat loaf in a recipe that will seem familiar to many in the more southern parts of Canada. The quail eggs are placed in the centre for visual interest, because as you slice into the loaf, you get a slice of egg.

2 lb	ground muskox	1 kg
2	eggs	2
3	cloves garlic, finely chopped	3
½ cup	fresh breadcrumbs	125 mL
1	10-oz/284-mL can onion soup, undiluted	1
½ tsp	salt	2 mL
1 tsp	freshly ground pepper	5 mL
4	quail eggs, hard-boiled and peeled	4
1 Tbsp	flour	15 mL
	Boiling water	

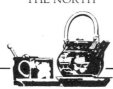

1. Preheat oven to 350°F/180°C.

2. Combine the ground meat, eggs, garlic, breadcrumbs, onion soup, salt and pepper and mix thoroughly.

3. Spread half the meat mixture in a loaf pan. Lay the quail eggs end to end in the centre of the meat. Add the rest of the meat, patting it around the eggs. Smooth the top of the meat loaf and bake for 1½ hours.

4. To unmould, run a knife around the edges of the meat loaf to loosen it from the pan. Invert the meat loaf onto a serving platter.

5. To make a gravy from the pan juices, pour off the excess fat from the loaf pan. Scrape all of the bits of flavoured meat from the sides and bottom of the pan. Place the pan on a burner over medium heat and add the flour, whisking it in to blend with the juices. Add boiling water, stirring constantly, to make approximately 1 cup/250 mL gravy. Simmer for a few minutes and taste for seasoning. Serve the gravy in a separate bowl.

Serves 4 to 6

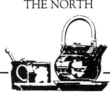

CARIBOU WITH PEPPERCORNS AND MUSTARD

Caribou is very lean and tender and it should be cooked on the rare side, like a very good piece of aged beef. Because it is so lean, it will require additional fat. You can lay strips of unsmoked bacon over the top as the meat is roasting, or marinate the meat in oil, as in this recipe.

¼ cup	soy sauce	50 mL
2 Tbsp	blueberry vinegar or other fruit vinegar	25 mL
½ cup	olive oil	125 mL
2 tsp	tarragon	10 mL
½ cup	crushed peppercorns	125 mL
4 lb	caribou roast, any cut	2 kg
¼ cup	dry mustard	50 mL

1. To make the marinade, combine the soy sauce, vinegar, oil, tarragon and half the peppercorns.

2. Coat the roast with the marinade, place in a glass dish and allow to marinate for 2 hours, turning every 20 minutes.

3. Preheat oven to 450°F/230°C.

4. Just before roasting, add the mustard and remaining peppercorns to the marinade to form a paste (add up to 1 Tbsp/15 mL more mustard if necessary). Using your hands, coat the roast as thoroughly as possible.

5. Roast for 15 minutes. Reduce heat to 325°F/160°C and continue roasting for 45 minutes to 1 hour. The roasting time will depend on the thickness of the roast (a roast about 2½ in/6 cm thick will require no more than 45 minutes if it is to be eaten rare).

6. Let the roast stand for 10 minutes before carving to allow the juices to flow back into the meat.

Serves 6

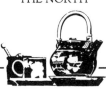

FLAT BASIL LOAVES

These are a summer specialty of the Alpine Bakery in Whitehorse. They can be eaten warm and fresh with butter or smeared with a tangy tomato sauce for an innovative pizza.

2½ cups	all-purpose flour	625 mL
1 tsp	salt	5 mL
1 cup	warm water	250 mL
1 Tbsp	olive oil	15 mL
1 tsp	Fermipan (instant yeast)	5 mL
¼ cup	finely chopped fresh basil or 1 Tbsp/ 15 mL dried basil	50 mL
1	egg, beaten	1
1 Tbsp	sesame or poppy seeds	15 mL

1. Combine 2 cups/500 mL flour with the salt. Stir in the water, oil and yeast until well mixed (if you can't find instant yeast, substitute 1 Tbsp/15 mL dry yeast, but proof it first in the warm water for 5 to 10 minutes).

2. Add the remaining flour, or until the dough is of a consistency to knead. Add more flour if necessary and knead for 8 to 10 minutes.

3. Oil the top of the dough and let it stand in a bowl in a warm place until double in bulk, about 45 minutes. Punch down the dough.

4. Sprinkle the basil on the work surface. Place the dough on top and knead, blending in the bits of herb.

5. Divide the dough into 6 pieces. Cover with a tea towel and let rise again until double in bulk. Punch down and flatten by hand.

6. Place the loaves on a buttered baking sheet and let them rise until almost double in bulk.

7. Preheat oven to 400°F/200°C. Indent the surface of the dough with your fingertips. Brush the surface with the beaten egg and sprinkle with sesame or poppy seeds. Bake for 15 to 20 minutes, or until golden and puffy.

Makes 6 flat loaves

—*Suat Tuzlak, Alpine Bakery, Whitehorse, Yukon*

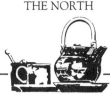

SOURDOUGH BREAD

You can shape this dough into the traditional round loaves or into crescent rolls, a French stick or dinner rolls. Vary the baking times accordingly. Sourdough bread is so basic in the North that people who have lived there for a long time are called Sourdoughs.

2½ cups	warm water	625 mL
1 cup	sourdough starter	250 mL
¼ cup	granulated sugar	50 mL
6 to 6½ cups	unbleached or all-purpose flour	1.5 to 1.6 L
¼ cup	melted butter	50 mL
2 tsp	salt	10 mL
2 Tbsp	cornmeal	25 mL

1. Combine the warm water, sourdough starter and sugar in a large, non-metallic bowl. Beat in 3 cups/750 mL flour.

2. Pour the melted butter over the dough to prevent it from drying out. Place the dough in a warm place for 4 to 6 hours or overnight.

3. After the dough has risen, stir it down and add the salt. Beat in the remaining flour a bit at a time until the dough loses its stickiness and can be kneaded. Knead for 8 to 10 minutes until it is smooth and elastic.

4. Divide the dough into 2 parts and shape into round loaves. Sprinkle a baking sheet with cornmeal. Place the loaves on the sheet.

5. Cover the loaves with a tea towel and let them rise in a warm place for 1½ hours.

6. Preheat oven to 400°F/200°C. Bake the loaves for 20 minutes, or until golden brown (the loaves should sound hollow when tapped).

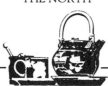

Sourdough Starter

Do not use a metal container or utensils for this recipe. It will give the dough an unpleasant flavour. You will need a large glass or enamelled bowl because the mixture will rise very high. When it collapses, the mixture may be transferred to a smaller glass bowl or jar.

1 Tbsp	dry yeast	15 mL
¼ cup	granulated sugar	50 mL
2 cups	unbleached or all-purpose flour	500 mL
2 cups	lukewarm water	500 mL

1. Combine the dry ingredients in a large, non-metallic bowl and stir in water. Allow the mixture to rise and recede. Transfer to a smaller container if desired.

2. Cover the mixture lightly and let it stand at room temperature for 3 to 5 days, stirring daily. When a clear, yellowish liquid accumulates on the top of the starter, it is ready to use. Refrigerate immediately.

3. Use the sourdough starter as required. This starter is designed to be used every 2 days. Replenish it as necessary (see below). If you can't use the starter all at once, it can be frozen. Thaw the starter and wait until it's bubbling before using.

4. To replenish the sourdough culture, combine 1½ cups/375 mL starter, 1 cup/250 mL milk, 1 cup/250 mL flour and ¼ cup/50 mL sugar. Mix and refrigerate as above. Wait 12 hours before using.

Makes 2 loaves

SOURDOUGH FLAPJACKS

Served generously as part of a Yukon breakfast (which also includes a mountain of eggs and ham or bacon) these pancakes provide enough strength to fight black bears. The batter must be started the night before. This recipe can also be doubled.

1 cup	unbleached or all-purpose flour	250 mL
1 cup	water	250 mL
½ cup	sourdough starter	125 mL
1 Tbsp	granulated sugar	15 mL
1	egg, slightly beaten	1
1 Tbsp	butter, melted	15 mL
¼ tsp	salt	1 mL
½ tsp	baking soda	2 mL

1. Combine the flour, water, sourdough starter and sugar in a large, non-metallic bowl, mixing until smooth. Let the mixture sit in a warm place overnight.

2. In the morning, mix together the egg, butter, salt and baking soda. Add to the flour mixture and stir until blended.

3. Lightly butter a hot skillet. Drop the dough by large spoonfuls onto the skillet and cook until the pancakes are covered with bubbles. Turn and cook until golden brown. Serve hot off the griddle with butter and lots of maple syrup.

Makes 12 pancakes

CHEESE BANNOCK

In Canada, bannock is associated with the Indians, though these round cakes are thought to have originated in Scotland. There are many variations on fat, flour and flavouring, and many recipes are designated for campfire or stove-top cooking.

This is a sophisticated bannock from Suat Tuzlak's Alpine Bakery in Whitehorse. It can be served instead of bread as part of a meal, as traditional bannock is, or it can be served at breakfast or tea with butter and fruit relish or jam. Either way, it is special.

½ cup	quick-cooking rolled oats	125 mL
½ cup	all-purpose flour	125 mL
1 cup	grated sharp Cheddar cheese	250 mL
pinch	salt	pinch
pinch	cayenne	pinch
¼ cup	butter	50 mL
¼ cup	water	50 mL

1. Preheat oven to 400°F/200°C.

2. Combine the rolled oats, flour, cheese, salt and cayenne.

3. With 2 knives or a pastry cutter, cut in the butter until the mixture has the texture of coarse meal.

4. Moisten the flour mixture with the water, mixing lightly with a fork until all the dough is dampened.

5. Gather the dough into a ball. Then flatten it with a rolling pin on a lightly floured surface. Roll into a rectangle, fold and roll again to ½-in/1-cm thickness.

6. Cut into 6 pieces, approximately 2 in × 4 in/5 cm × 10 cm.

7. Place on an ungreased baking sheet. Bake for 10 to 12 minutes, or until golden brown. Serve warm.

Makes 6 bannock

—Suat Tuzlak, Alpine Bakery, Whitehorse, Yukon

INDEX